True You

a Journey to Finding and Loving Yourself

True You

Janet Jackson

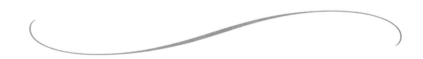

with DAVID RITZ

afterword by DAVID ALLEN

GALLERY
BOOKS

Gallery Books / Karen Hunter Publishing
PUBLISHED BY SIMON & SCHUSTER
New York   London   Toronto   Sydney

Gallery Books
A Division of Simon & Schuster, Inc.
1230 Avenue of the Americas
New York, NY 10020

Karen Hunter Publishing
A Division of Suitt-Hunter Enterprises, LLC
P.O. Box 632
South Orange, NJ 07079

First Karen Hunter Publishing/Gallery Books hardcover edition February 2011

GALLERY BOOKS and colophon are registered trademarks of Simon & Schuster, Inc.

For information about special discounts for bulk purchases,
please contact Simon & Schuster Special Sales at 1-866-506-1949
or business@simonandschuster.com.

The Simon & Schuster Speakers Bureau can bring authors to your live event.
For more information or to book an event contact the Simon & Schuster Speakers
Bureau at 1-866-248-3049 or visit our website at www.simonspeakers.com.

Designed by Joy O'Meara

Manufactured in the United States of America

10   9   8   7   6   5   4   3   2   1

Library of Congress Cataloging-in-Publication Data

Jackson, Janet
    True you / Janet Jackson; with David Ritz. — 1st Karen Hunter Publishing/
Pocket Books hardcover ed.
        p.   cm.
    1. Jackson, Janet.   2. Singers—United States—Biography.
I. Ritz, David.   II. Title.
    ML420.J153A3   2011
    782.42166092—dc22
    [B]   2010039261

ISBN 978-1-4165-8724-8
ISBN 978-1-4516-3604-8 (ebook)

Acknowledgments

Writing my first book was an adventure, and each acknowledgment comes from my heart with love.

To my fans, because sharing your stories with me in person, in letters, and on-line gave me the courage to tell my own. So many of you taught me that you needed to be heard. I hope you recognize your voices and that you realize I understand, I care, and I love you. Thank you for loving me, no matter what.

David Ritz, my co-author, we've been talking about doing something for years. We finally made it happen and I am grateful to you. Karen Hunter, for passion and patience.

My nutritionist, David Allen. Chef Andre of A Café and Chris Strong, both from Kathy Ireland Worldwide, for recipes and tasty food. These recipes are real. We enjoyed them over and over again.

Thank you to Mother and my entire family.

I give thanks to Jesus Christ, who leads me and protects me every day.

My jdj Entertainment management team, Jaime Mendoza, Jessica Davenport because you're always there, and Terri Harris because you're you. Joey Maldonado, Lucy Reyes. My Sterling Winters Company management team, Jason Winters, my godfather, Erik Sterling, Stephen Roseberry, Jon Carrasco.

Acknowledgments

"Grant," Lynnette Bowers, and everyone at Grant, Tani, Barash, and Altman. Tom Hoberman, Seth Lichtenstein, and Adam Kaller at Hansen, Hoberman, Jacobson and Klein. John Marx, Charles King, Ari Emmanuel, and everyone at WME.

Fran Cooper, Robert Behar, Janet Zeitoun for trying to keep it a little bit cute. Gil Duldulao for dances, dreams, and friendship.

Tony Martinez for making me laugh, while making me sweat myself into shape. Everyone can't have the luxury of a fitness genius to train them. I'm so fortunate to have you and I would not have been able to write this book without you. I want to share your gifts with the world.

My musicians, dancers, singers, and entire tech concert crew.

To Simon & Schuster and Karen Hunter Publishing (Charles Suitt and Karen Hunter) for publishing this book.

This is not an autobiography. It's a journey that I am still taking to love and to accept myself just as I am. I want you to walk this road with me. You can never be happy until you understand why you're doing what you're doing. If this book helps people find those answers, it has succeeded.

Finally, this is for you, you know who you are and you know why I love you. I'm glad we waited for what we have now.

Love,
Janet

Follow Janet at http://www.janetjackson.com, Twitter, Facebook, and MySpace.

To Mike

Contents

True You

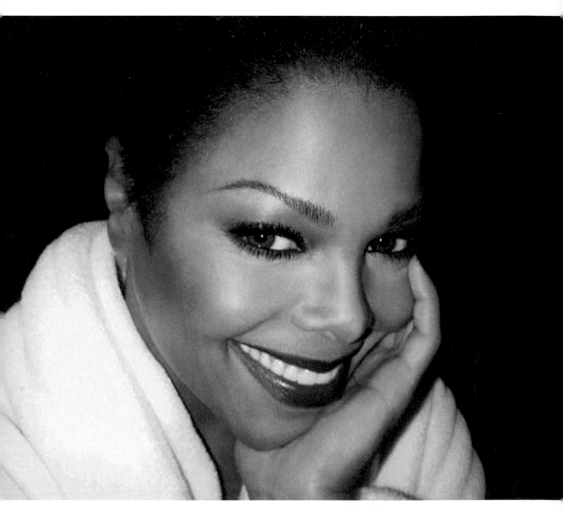

At home after a day of shooting *For Colored Girls*.

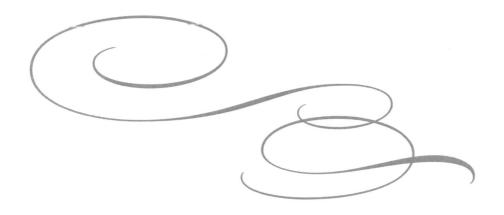

Breaking Free

In 1977, at age ten, I was cast on the TV sitcom *Good Times*. My character was Penny, an abused child in desperate need of love. I really didn't want to do the show. I didn't want to be away from my family. And being on television only added to my negative feelings about my body.

Before production began, I was told two things: I was fat and needed to slim down, and because I was beginning to develop, I needed to bind my breasts. In both cases the message was devastating—my body was wrong. The message was also clear—to be successful, I had to change the way I looked.

I didn't even know what it meant to "bind my breasts." At first I was frightened. Were they talking about some kind of operation? For a girl so young, this was confusing. Naturally, I kept the confusion to myself.

"It means we need to tie down your breasts so you appear flat-chested," the wardrobe woman explained.

So, each day of shooting, I went through the ordeal of having wide strips of gauze tied across my chest to hide the natural shape of my breasts. It was uncomfortable and humiliating.

I never discussed this with anyone. Never said a word to my parents, sisters, or brothers. I kept it all hidden inside. I didn't know what to do with my feelings of fear and embarrassment. So I hid them. I was ashamed of them. After all, I was an actress, and my job was to please others—writers, directors, and producers—and to entertain the audience. There was no room for personal confusion.

Had there been a book that addressed issues like body image, I would have read it immediately. Had there been a book that told me I wasn't alone—that millions of men, women, and children are confused about self-image—I would have been grateful. That kind of book could have made a difference in my life.

I want this book to make a difference.

It's important that I present myself just as I am. So I must tell you right away that I'm no expert. I have no psychic powers and I sure don't possess any secret wisdom. I'm just Janet. I have strengths, weaknesses, fears, happiness, sadness. I experience joy and I experience pain. I'm highly emotional. I'm very vulnerable. And, as anyone who knows me well will testify, I'm extremely sensitive. I have lifelong patterns of behavior that have caused me difficulty—patterns tough to break. Like everyone, I have talents, but with those talents have come challenges.

This book is about meeting the challenges that face all of us.

For more than three decades, I've struggled with yo-yo dieting. Some of my battles with weight have been very public. But most of them have been internal. Even at my thinnest, when my body was being praised, I wasn't happy with what I saw in the mirror or how I felt about myself.

I've never talked about the origins of my up-and-down struggles until now, but they started at a very young age. I've also never discussed the crazy rumors that have swirled around me—that, for example, I've had ribs removed and other extreme plastic surgery. It makes me angry to read those lies, but I've never bothered to reply.

I've never gone into the hard work involved in getting myself—mind and spirit, heart and soul—into shape. I've waited for the right time, and have decided that that time is now.

It has taken me most of my adult life to come to terms with who I am. To do that, I had to break free of attitudes that brought me down. I had to set and meet realistic goals. I had to eat better, exercise better, look better, feel better, be better.

But how?

When self-esteem seems like nothing more than a concept you hear about on talk shows, how do you make it real? How do you start feeling good about yourself when feeling bad has been a life-long pattern? How do you go from feeling unworthy—a condition I know as well as anyone—to feeling useful? How do you make the transition from being unrelentingly self-critical to generously self-accepting?

I want to share with you stories from my own struggles. But I also want to share stories I've been privileged to hear—from fans and friends who have dealt with the same issues. I believe these stories will help you.

I'm an optimist. I know we can change. Problems, even the most severe ones, can be solved. We can be happy with who we are. Whether we're a size two or twenty, whether we're tall, short, narrow, or wide, we can learn to love those things about our-selves that are truly beautiful—the things that come from within and matter the most.

At the deepest level, we're all related, and we all can relate. We *need* to relate to survive the emotional storms that come our way. I hope this book can, in whatever small way, help you weather those storms.

I've been writing this book in some form for most of my adult life. The journey to arrive at a place of knowing and loving myself has been long and hard.

I'm not surprised when I'm asked, "How can you—of all people—have self-esteem issues?" But please believe me: my struggles are real.

I'm grateful for success. Success is wonderful. The truth, though, is that being in the spotlight can complicate personal problems even more. You never have a chance to deal with yourself privately and work through issues on your own. Everything is on display for the world to see. My pattern has been depressingly clear: fear and uncertainty lead to feeling bad about myself. Bad feelings lead to depression, and depression leads to overeating. Food is my escape and my comfort. It started that way at a young age and has remained a constant. When I fall into a funk, I turn to food. At some point I learned to control my eating, especially when I had something to do—for example, a record, concert, or TV appearance. I had the ability to work out, stay on a strict regimen, and make it happen. I stayed disciplined.

In 2006, when I gained weight for a film and blew up to 180 pounds, pictures of me appeared in the tabloids. Only my closest friends knew that I was still running in the sand every day from three to five miles. I was big. I was muscular. I was strong. I wasn't eating pizza. I was exercising. I was heavier than I wanted to be, but I was not weak. Losing that additional ten or fifteen pounds, though, seemed impossible, in spite of my workouts.

So my heart goes out to people who say they work out but still can't lose weight—or who eat very little and yet can't slim down. I know the frustration. I know the sadness.

I also know that sexism enters into the picture: mass and muscle is considered sexy on men. But women are judged by harsher standards; they are often unrealistic and unfair.

When I was diligently trying to lose this excessive weight

through exercise, few understood what was happening. Even the editor of this book was stunned to learn that during this period I was vigorously working out.

Because the production company changed the dates, my other commitments forced me to cancel the film. I was deeply disappointed. I was really ready for this role. In one scene my character had to go in the water wearing just her underwear. I was willing to do that. I wanted people to see that I put craft as an actor above glamour and image.

I spent so much time psychologically preparing for this role that when it fell through I looked up and didn't recognize myself. I wasn't just plump; I was fat. My stomach got in the way of tying my shoes. My feet and joints ached when I stepped out of bed in the morning. Because none of my clothes fit, I lived in sweats. I stayed in sweats because I refused to buy more clothes; this was not the size I planned on staying at.

I knew it was bad when one day I jumped up onto my kitchen counter to sit, as I would often do, and felt excruciating pain in my side. That simple, ordinary movement was beyond my ability.

I realized that this would be my greatest weight challenge. I had to drop weight, but how?

Discipline.

But discipline wasn't enough. I said to myself, "You can do this. You've done things that are harder than this."

I started running even more. And what normally worked for me—extreme working out and extreme dieting—just wasn't cutting it.

That was when I decided to get help. I admitted that I couldn't do it alone.

I eventually lost the weight. And in the process, I learned many things about myself. I learned that the weight gain and the inability to lose it didn't involve just a role in a movie. It wasn't just a one-time event—because honestly, I had been having this battle my entire life.

The journey to self-understanding surpassed my desire to be a certain size or a certain weight.

As I went through this tremendous weight-loss challenge, I thought to myself, *Others have had this same struggle. I need to share mine.* That has led me to this book.

My goal is to make it easier for anyone—girl, woman, boy, or man—dealing with the things I dealt with.

In 2008, I lost the sixty pounds but gained something far more valuable: a love and appreciation for myself that I will never lose.

My hope and prayer is that my story, and others' as well, will help you turn *your story* in a positive and loving direction.

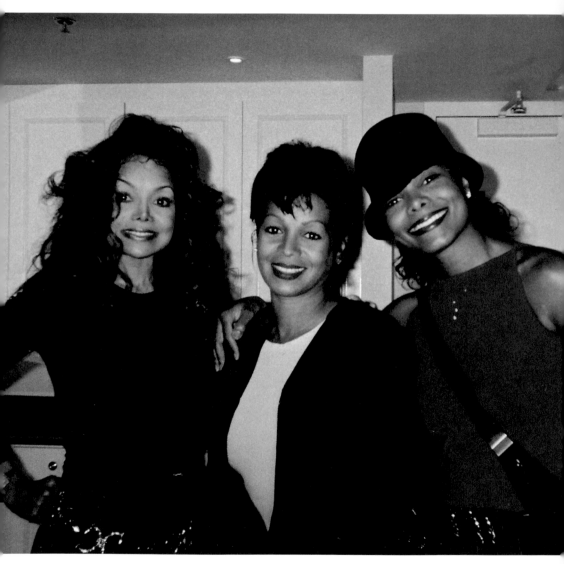

During the All for You tour in Hawaii with my sisters.

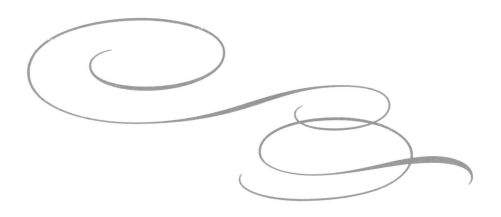

"As Pretty as . . . ."

Where do our feelings of being less-than come from? Why does emotional insecurity seem to follow us from the very start of our lives?

If we're going to figure that out, it might be helpful to go back to the beginning. The oldest stories are sometimes the most telling.

My earliest memories are of growing up in an enormous English Tudor home in suburban Encino, California, just outside Los Angeles. I was born in Gary, Indiana, but I have only one distinct memory from there: the marriage of my sister Rebbie. I recall much love and warmth from that day. It is after my brothers become famous and we move to California, though, that my memories really kick in.

I was a different kind of kid. The sadness of a gloomy rainy day made me happy. The sound and smell of rain relaxed me. I loved the ping-ping-ping of raindrops against my window. I'd ask Mother if she could take me in her car for a ride in the rain. Later in life, when I had my license, I'd spend hours driving through rainstorms.

I liked the mood of a gray sky. I liked leaning against the window and gazing at the wet world outside. I liked the connection to water. When it came time to choosing bedrooms, I chose the one in the north wing. It faced one of my favorite features of the house, an elaborate fountain that sat at the entrance of the long cobblestone driveway. I loved listening to the water cascading out of the fountain. Falling water eased my mind.

One day when I was six, I awoke early and saw that the rain, which had begun the night before, was still coming down. It was a gentle rain, a rare Southern California summer storm. I ran outside just to feel it on my face. I didn't mind getting my hair wet in the rain. I liked it. As a little girl, I wore my hair in braids. I only started combing it when I began to perform. Getting my hair soaked in a downpour felt like freedom.

Back inside, I dried off and went to the family library. The books that lined the walls gave the room a stillness that I loved.

I also loved the warmth of the room—the heat was turned up high. Heat keeps me calm.

At the end of the library was a huge picture window with a sill large enough to accommodate me. I could stretch out and read on my stomach, or my back, or sit up with my legs crossed. Sometimes I would fall asleep there. Other times I would just stare out at the pouring rain.

On this particular afternoon, I happened to notice a framed picture of my sister Rebbie, taken when she had graduated from high school. Without a doubt, she was the most beautiful girl I had ever seen. At that moment, this thought came to me: *When I grow up, will I ever be as pretty as Rebbie?* That's what I was hoping for. I know that I genuinely admired my sister's beauty, but looking back I can also see that by comparing myself to her, I felt inadequate.

It would have been wonderful to have someone say to me, "Don't compare yourself to anyone else. Comparisons are almost always harmful. Comparisons mean there's a winner and loser—and you're the one who winds up feeling like a loser."

This book is about finding the true you and knowing you're beautiful as you are. Forget the ugly messages of comparison. I remember those comparisons when I was the only black child in an all-white school. Some of the kids did things that weren't intended to be mean, but they were funky and made me feel less-than. I remember them wanting to touch my hair because it wasn't straight—it was different.

Just the other day, I thought about comparisons when a friend told me this story:

A mother walked into the bedroom of her five-year-old daughter. The little girl, scissors in hand, was busy snipping all the curls off her very curly hair.

"Baby!" cried the mother. "What are you doing?"

"Getting pretty," said the little girl. "All the pretty girls in my school have straight hair."

"You *are* pretty," said the mother. "Curls *are* pretty."

"But straight hair is prettier. With straight hair, I'll be more popular and everyone will love me."

The story broke my heart.

And yet we all have similar stories.

As a little kid, I almost immediately started judging myself against others. That convinced me that something was missing. I felt that I was the wrong size and the wrong shape.

When we are kids, so many of us feel that things are wrong—not wrong with the world, but *wrong with us.*

We're not smart. We're not valuable. We're not worthy of being loved.

We're also unable to stop idealizing others and minimizing ourselves.

He's taller.

She's thinner.

He's cooler.

She's prettier.

How do we break free of that way of thinking? What do we do when those voices—powerful and persistent negative voices—have us believing in everything but ourselves?

The truth of the matter is this:

The true you *is* curly hair.

The true you *is* straight hair.

The true you *is* kinky hair, blond hair, black hair, and every shade in between.

Everyone is different, and beautifully unique.

If we value our uniqueness, we value everything about us. We don't need to look for a model of perfect beauty when we realize that our own beauty can't be duplicated.

At age six, though, I didn't have the slightest clue about my uniqueness. All I knew was that my sister was the most beautiful woman in the world—and I'd never come close to her beauty. By age six, I was already feeling bad about myself.

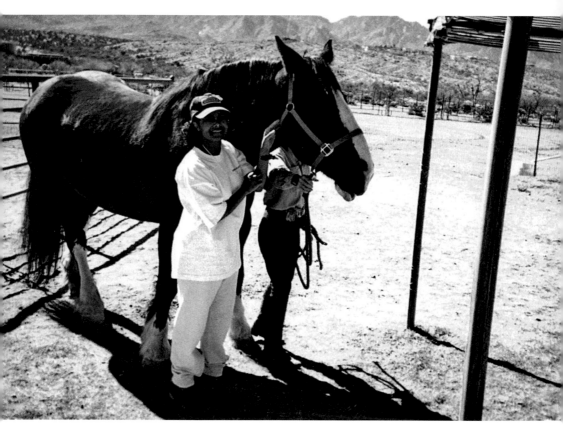

I've always loved horses, even though I'm somewhat allergic to them. If they're not absolutely clean, I break out in hives. That doesn't stop me from riding and loving them anyway. In Arizona, soul searching. Knowing I was looking for something and not understanding what it was. This was a period of healing and a beginning step, asking questions about myself that have brought me to where I am today.

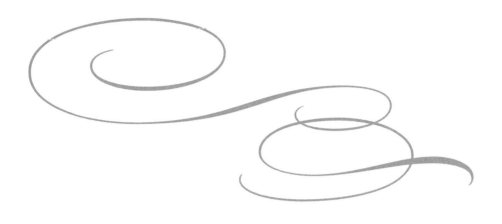

Hold Back the Tears

I deeply believe the words that Marvin Gaye wrote: *we're all sensitive people.*

My own sensitivity became evident to me when, early in my life, my brothers started teasing me. There was nothing unusual about that, of course. Most brothers tease their sisters—and vice versa. When we remember the taunting words as adults, though, the teasing sounds malicious. But it's simply part of childhood. It's how sisters and brothers relate to each other.

My brother Mike teased me the most. I adored Mike, and I know he adored me. We were extremely close. Whether it was because I was the baby of the family, or because we were kindred souls, Mike and I understood each other on a deep and loving level. He had a beautiful heart. From the very beginning of my life, I was inspired by his talent. That continues to this day.

But even with our strong connection, there was a great deal of teasing on Michael's part. He had all sorts of names for me. For example, he called me "Dunk." I think that came from "donkey." I actually cherish the name today because it was his gift to me. A lot of his pet names had to do with my backside. I don't cherish those names as much. But teasing was part of Mike's humor. He meant no harm.

He often told me that I needed to be thinner. He had a vision of how I should look. When we went to the roller rink, he pointed out a girl who, in his view, had an ideal figure. To protect her privacy, I'll call her Andy. Andy was white and svelte. She had a petite backside. As I got to know her, I learned she rode horses, and soon horseback riding became a passion of mine. In my eyes, Andy was perfect. She proudly displayed the ribbons she had won in equestrian competitions. She was well-dressed and well-mannered. I guess part of me wanted to be Andy.

When my brothers went riding, I held my breath until they invited me. I didn't have the nerve to invite myself. When I wasn't asked to come along, I was crushed. When I was asked, I was elated. Every time I rode, I broke out in hives, but didn't care. I loved the sport. And even though I looked up to the ladylike Andy, I was a natural tomboy. I liked climbing trees with my brothers. I liked wearing T-shirts and jeans. I fantasized about driving trucks and jeeps.

Girls and women have a special relationship to jeans. At least *I* always have. When I reached age eight, I started wearing Dittos, as many of the other girls were doing. It was hard finding pants that fit me well. I was small in the waist but round in the rear. Dittos' Saddlebacks accentuated my behind. I owned a pair of Saddlebacks but was too self-conscious to wear them in public. I probably looked fine in Saddlebacks; I might have even looked cute. But I had internalized my brother's teasing. I was convinced that my body shape was terribly wrong.

Later in life, even after I thought I had gotten over my complex about having a big butt, I remember checking into a hotel and using the name "Andy" to ensure my privacy. Then it hit me: why of all names should I have chosen "Andy"? At that moment I realized that I still had not let go of the Andy I knew; I still saw her as some fantasy, the perfect woman with the perfect body.

The things that get us early in life and stay with us!

Being teased. Being sensitive. Comparing ourselves to others.

All of those things can come together in powerful ways, as in a story a friend recently told me.

As a little boy, my friend had a severe stutter. He hated going to school. When the teacher called on him for an answer, he couldn't get out a word. The teacher presumed he didn't know the answer. The other kids teased him unmercifully, comparing him to Porky

Pig. He was taken out of an advanced class and put into a slow class. That only made him stutter more. His frustrations mounted. The greater his frustration, the worse his stutter, and the more the other kids laughed.

He told his mother that he didn't want to go to school. She asked why, but he wouldn't say. He kept his feelings inside. Inside he felt that, compared to the other kids with their fluent speech, he was nobody.

His mom insisted that he return to school, but things there got even worse. His teachers grew more impatient, his fellow students crueler. One night he finally told his mother what was wrong. His stutter was a source of tremendous shame.

"All the teasing makes me want to die," he said. "Don't make me go back to school," he begged.

"You have to go to school," she insisted.

He broke down crying, and the next morning, when he refused to go to school, his father took him there by force, dragging him into the classroom. The other kids pointed at him and laughed. My friend remembers this as the most humiliating moment of his life.

As an adult, though, my friend recognizes this as a moment when his parents were expressing love. They knew that sooner or later he'd have to face school. He'd have to face the world. They couldn't protect him from that, and love required that they take action. They also sent him to a speech therapist. That, too, was part of their love.

Today my friend can still feel the pain of that humiliation, but it's the love that saw him through. He made it through the challenge of those early years, He still stutters, but the stutter doesn't stop him from speaking, even in public situations.

"My stutter is part of me," he says. "I'm not interested in hiding it or even losing it. As long as it doesn't control me, I'm fine. As long as it doesn't keep me from doing what I want to do and saying what I want to say, I'm a happy stutterer."

When I ask my friend what practical solution he found most helpful, he explains it this way: "Put the problem—whatever it is—out there. Be open about it. Discuss it. Keep a journal. Record your thoughts and fears. Tell a friend. Tell your parents, and if they're not sympathetic, tell an aunt or an uncle, a grandma or grandpa. Don't try and hide. Fear thrives in isolation. Once exposed to the light of day, its power fades. The best advice I got about stuttering applies to many problems associated with shame. I was told to *intentionally* stutter in new situations, even when I didn't have to. The speech therapist said, 'When you try to pretend you're not a stutterer and struggle to be fluent, you get even more nervous. So in any new situation, stutter on your first words. From the get-go, let people know that you're a stutterer. You have nothing to hide, nothing to be ashamed of. If people laugh, that's their problem. Just be who you are.' "

The true you.

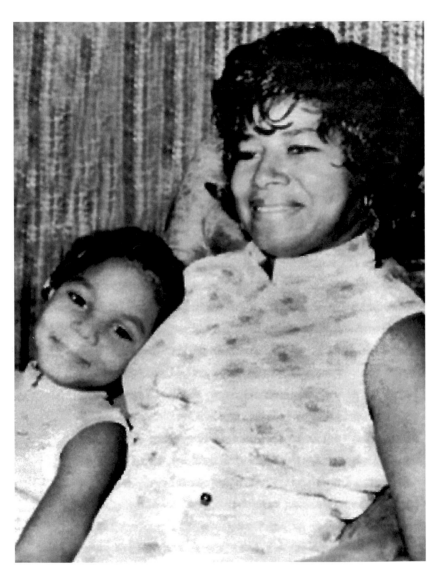

Mother's love.

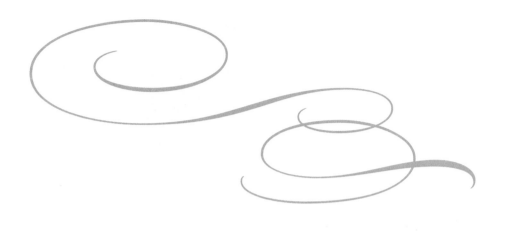

"I'll Just Starve Myself"

Mike's teasing really got to me. I took it way too seriously. But the more he joked about my big behind, the more determined I was to be thin. Even as a little kid. On certain days I decided simply to starve myself—no breakfast, no lunch. Because ours was a show business family, we were pretty much on our own. Other than the extremely rare holiday dinner, we didn't have regular sit-down meals.

There were times when Mother cooked marvelous meals. As a little girl, I loved everything she prepared. There was a special connection between us. She told me that I was the most affectionate of her children, the one who went around kissing my siblings and telling them "I love you." I'm sure I was just mirroring my mother.

Even though Mother was very busy helping her children with their personal lives, she always found time to cook. The refrigerator was packed with whatever we wanted, and we could eat as much and as often as we liked.

That's why I decided early on—without really thinking about it—that I had to depend upon my own willpower to lose weight. It was a matter of determination. Most of the kids in our neighborhood were Jewish, so there were always platters of bagels and cream cheese around, even at school. I love bagels and cream cheese. If I ate only a bite, though, I'd force myself to skip lunch. I'd get through the afternoon, but by the time I got home I was starving.

I had to break down and fix myself something to eat. I wasn't tall enough to reach the stove, so I'd grab a stool, climb up, swivel around, reach in the freezer, and bring out a good-sized steak. I'd watched my siblings do it, I'd watch Mother, and I was determined to do it, too. I'd thaw out the meat, tenderize it, slice up the onions, go heavy on the salt and pepper, and butter up the pan. With jerking motions, I'd swivel all the way back so I could face the oven and stick that puppy inside. I loved watching it cook. The smells were intoxicating. When it was ready, *I* was ready. Nothing has ever tasted that good.

Sometimes after school I'd go with friends to their homes. I was amazed that they were not allowed to raid the refrigerator. Their moms left precise instructions with the housekeeper about what could and could not be consumed by the kids. That seemed so strange to me—they actually had to *ask* for food.

Meanwhile, I was consuming whatever I liked, and I liked almost everything. And because our household was run on the unspoken principle of self-reliance, I kept relying on my own cooking instincts.

Paradoxically, I loved to eat but felt that I didn't deserve to eat. The name-calling made me self-conscious about my size, and so I fell into that same pattern.

In my crazy head I heard that old familiar voice saying, "You're fat. You've got to move away from food. You shouldn't eat a thing."

That voice led to a skimpy lunch or no lunch.

A school friend's father owned a chain of McDonald's. After a field trip, our entire class went to their home and were surprised with food from one of their stores. You can't imagine how excited I was. I knew the food was fattening, but I couldn't pass up a hot Big Mac and french fries. It meant I could be like the rest of the kids in my class. I ate the hamburger and fries; I drank a milk shake. I felt normal; I felt good. But the next day I was back to skipping lunch at school.

By the time I got home I was famished and wound up staring at a huge sweet potato pie.

First voice: "Eat it."

Second voice: "Don't touch it."

First voice: "You know you want it."

Second voice: "You know you're fat."

First voice: "You know how good it'll taste."

Second voice: "You know how you'll get fatter."

First voice: "Fatter doesn't matter."

Second voice: "The fatter, the uglier."

First voice: "You'll never be as pretty as Rebbie, so you might as well eat the pie."

Second voice: "Resist."

First voice: "Give in."

Second voice: "Don't."

First voice: "Do."

I did.

I ate the majority of the delicious pie. I was stuck in an argument between two voices that I couldn't win. The result was a feeling of emotional defeat. I lost.

Food was an enemy, food was a friend, food was comfort. And often that comfort came in the form of the person preparing the food, whether it be mother or my grandmother.

I had a strong emotional connection to my grandmother Crystal Lee. We called her Grandmama, and she was extraordinary. She carried a big smile and a mouth full of teeth. We always knew when she arrived because her voice bounced off the walls. You could hear her from the other end of the block. Even our parrot would start screaming "Grandma!" the minute she walked in.

We had housekeepers who were good cooks. As I said, Mother was a superb cook, but when Grandmama was around, she ruled. The kitchen was her kingdom, and you were lucky if she asked you to help. There was food everywhere, all made from scratch—apple pie, blueberry cobbler, peach cobbler. You name it.

Jermaine liked German chocolate cake and pineapple upside-down cake, so Grandmama and Mother made sure to have them on hand. Mike liked carrot cake, and so that was definitely on the menu, too. Grandmama made the best liver and onions. I was the kind of kid who ate anything and everything—candied yams, Cornish hens, greens with ham hocks, salmon croquettes, deep-fried catfish, deep-fried chicken, turkey chili, black-eyed peas, pinto beans. Grandmama cooked in the Southern style, as did Mother, who came from Alabama, as well as my father, who came from Arkansas.

All this meant mountains of sugar, tons of butter, and oceans of salt. Sitting on that swivel stool, watching Grandmama cook, I took it all in—and helped. I loved chopping the vegetables, kneading the dough, and baking the biscuits. As I helped, I sampled everything.

Food made me feel great. Food was the symbol and substance of the care being offered; food was everything warm and wonderful.

Grandmama not only cared enough to feed me, but was also patient enough to teach me to cook. We all fooled around in the kitchen. My father liked to roast peanuts, and Mike, Randy, and I made caramel apples and ice cream.

Grandmama laid the foundation for me in the kitchen.

Again, it was the push and pull. Those internal voices fighting against one another, together with my already twisted view of myself and my beauty, led me down the wrong path in terms of body image and self-esteem.

Maybe it was the teasing, maybe it was that sense of perfectionism that gets ingrained in so many kids—but whatever it was, I got the message early: I was chubby. I was bloated. I had curves in the wrong places. My body was out of whack. It's strange, but when I look back at my kid pictures, I don't see an overweight little girl. I look perfectly normal. But the word *normal* was never used to describe me. I didn't feel normal. I felt fat.

My friend who stutters remembers that he felt stupid because others—his classmates and even some of his teachers—associated his impediment with a dimwit. He saw the world as nearly all children do: through the eyes of others. My opinion of myself—even my literal vision of myself—was determined by how I *thought* others perceived me. I emphasize "thought" because I really didn't know. My brother Mike may not have seen me as fat; he was just teasing. But I took his teasing to heart. I embraced it, internalized it, and, without knowing it, became tormented by it for years to come.

Kids are easily injured. Kids are sensitive. Kids keep secrets. I kept my feelings of inadequacy from everyone, so there was no way my parents could have reassured me and told me I was fine the way I was, that I didn't have to reshape my body or conform to an image that the white culture found acceptable. But my parents, God bless them, had tremendous challenges of their own. They had worked tirelessly to keep nine kids off the street, feed them, educate them, and develop their natural talents. My parents were overwhelmed with responsibilities. They had to nurture their instinctive strategies for survival, a work ethic for themselves and their children. My parents were about discipline, focus, and, in the case of my mother, extraordinary loving care.

I identify with children, teens, young adults, with anyone whose parents, no matter how loving, don't have the psychological insight to help them through their crises. If we have an understanding sibling, an uncle, an aunt, a grandmother, a surrogate mom or dad who can reassure us that we don't have to measure up to someone else's standard—that's beautiful. If we don't have such a person in our lives, my hope is that we can find that voice deep inside us, a voice that lets us know that we are who we are. Different. Unique. Worthwhile. God's child.

We don't need to compare. We just need to be.

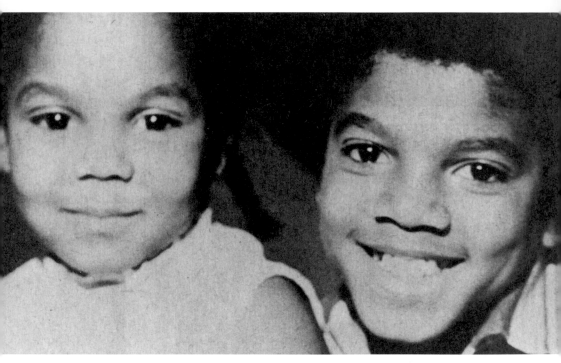

With my beloved big brother Mike.

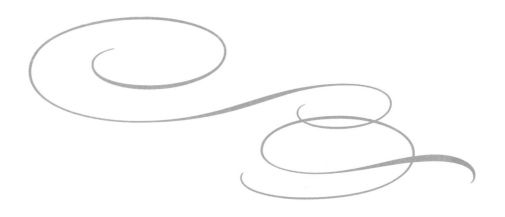

"Smile, though your heart
is aching / Smile, even
though it's breaking."

At the memorial service for Michael, my brother Jermaine
sang "Smile," a song written by Charlie Chaplin and beloved the
world over. Jermaine sang it beautifully. Mike loved the song, too,
and recorded an exquisite version of it. "Smile" resonates with all

the Jackson children, because it captures not only the sweetness of music—and music's power to heal—but also the obligation we have always felt as entertainers, from the earliest age, to place the audience's need to be entertained above whatever pain we might be experiencing.

I can't describe our pain in losing our brother, or the pain of his children in losing their father, or the pain of my parents in losing their son. I still have not seen the film *This Is It*. I still can't watch any of his videos or listen to his music. I'm certain that one day I'll again be able to enjoy the miraculous sound of his voice and the marvelous sight of his dancing, but that day has not yet arrived. The mourning continues.

As Jermaine sang "Smile," I thought it was the perfect anthem to remember our brother by. Michael made us smile, even when his heart was breaking.

I, too, was taught to always smile, and yet, ironically, most of my life I never liked my smile. It felt fraudulent. I smiled not because I was happy but because I adopted the message of the song that said "Light up your face with gladness, / Hide every trace of sadness."

I remember seeing Jack Nicholson as the Joker in *Batman* and thinking, *Wow, when he smiles I can see all the way to the back of his throat. That's what my smile looks like. My smile is hideous.* Because I didn't like my full smile, I often just grinned. In contrast to Grandmama's beautiful smile, my smile felt forced.

Later in life, my friend and producer Jimmy Jam was at a video shoot of mine. Things weren't going well, and I expressed my anxiety.

"I understand, Janet," said Jimmy. "But forget the problems and just smile."

"Why would I do that?" I asked. "My smile is not my best feature."

"What!" Jimmy countered. "Are you crazy? People *love* your smile."

"They do?"

"No one's ever told you that?"

"No."

"Well, I'm telling you. Smile, girl. Just smile."

My siblings and I grew up with the belief that you don't let people know what is going on inside. We didn't carry our problems onstage. Fans paid hard-earned money to watch us perform, and our job was to make them happy. End of story.

My early life as a performer was rooted in this unspoken belief—suppress your feelings.

As a child, I shot an ad for Disney. They put me in Mouseketeer ears and asked me to smile. I did. I haven't seen that photograph since, and my sincere hope is that it has disappeared forever.

That day, because I was missing schoolwork, I was given a tutor. At the time I was not in the advanced reading group at school, and so I had a bit of a complex about it. I loved to read, but was never a fast reader. In contrast, I saw my siblings as brilliant students who always got top grades. When my mother was in school, she had earned straight A's. I felt inadequate. And even though as a small child I dreamed of going to college, I was afraid that I was not college material. How could I ever comprehend books that were two or three hundred pages long? I expressed my fears to the tutor, who in turn told my mother.

Mother was upset that I had confided in a stranger. My confession may well have embarrassed her. Mother is a proud and private woman who feels that whatever is happening within the family should remain within the family. I apologized for talking too openly to the tutor. Again, I learned my lesson, but at what cost?

I felt bad, because I wanted so very much to please my mother—and I hadn't. She was justifiably proud that her young daughter had been chosen to do this advertisement. I had competed against hundreds of other kids, and I had succeeded. Why couldn't I just be happy with that success and keep whatever confusion I might have been feeling to myself? From then on, I vowed that I would do just that.

My need to please others was immense and I suspect that the same is true for most kids. Whether we're competing to be in an advertisement, or participating in a spelling bee or beauty contest, we want to win, not so much for ourselves but for others, and especially our parents.

We don't know that love is something that already exists within; we act like it has to be earned. Our attitude: *If we give pleasure to others, we'll get love for ourselves.* But except for those brief moments when the world awards us, that approach makes us miserable.

When I first started performing at age seven, I had silently accepted that my duty was to please others. Naturally, I would enter into the family business, where my brothers had succeeded on a spectacular level. Although it was never stated, the same degree of success was expected of me.

My brother Mike helped prepare me with my lines, my singing, and my little dance routine. My brother Randy was my partner. We were part of the show at the MGM in Las Vegas. We pretended to be an adult couple. Randy was Sonny and I was dressed up like Cher. We sang "I Got You Babe" and at the end, I was handed a black doll to represent their daughter Chastity. In another skit, I wore a gown and struck a sexy pose like Mae West, mouthing her famous line, "Why don't you come up and see me sometime?" The audience howled.

The standing ovation we received every night let me know that I had done my job.

I absorbed the audience's appreciation, recognition, and love. It all felt good. It felt especially good to be part of my family and contributing to the creativity that made us special.

It was a mixed blessing, but a blessing nonetheless. To be close with one's siblings is a beautiful thing. It's comfort, it's reassurance, it's security. I have great memories of that togetherness, and though at times I yearned for what seemed a more "normal" childhood, I didn't see my life as a young entertainer as being especially rigorous or hard. It was all I knew.

For example, Mike and I loved to re-create dance steps that we watched from the golden age of Hollywood—moves perfected by Gene Kelly and Cyd Charisse, Fred Astaire and Ginger Rogers. By the side of our pool, we'd also mimic the moves of fabulous tap dancers such as the Nicholas Brothers. I didn't see this as work; I saw it as a fun. And when it was time to go to work, I was ready.

Once, just before a Jackson Family TV special in which Randy and I were scheduled to perform "Yes, Sir, That's My Baby," I came down with chicken pox. I felt ill physically, but I felt even worse emotionally. I was worried to death that I wouldn't get to go on. How could I miss the show? If I didn't perform, Randy would also be deprived of performing. How could I do that to my brother? How could I let him down? Fortunately, I got well just in time and, wearing a blue dress with a boa at the top, I strolled out in front of the cameras and we did our thing.

It was exciting to perform onstage, but just as exciting were those brief moments when I got to live the life of a normal child.

One day after school a friend invited me to a Brownie troop meeting. I was dying to see what the Brownies were all about, and I gladly accepted. At the home of one of our classmates, they had a little arts and crafts project. They all wore their little uniforms. They planned outings—a trip to Disneyland, a hike in the hills, a visit to an old-age home to cheer up the elderly. I yearned to wear a Brownie uniform and join the troop, but there was no way that could happen. My performance schedule wouldn't allow it.

Mother was angry when I arrived home late from the Brownie meeting. I hadn't asked permission to go. She didn't know where I was and so was understandably worried. I apologized. I didn't tell her how badly I wanted to be a Brownie. I didn't explain how much I loved being at the meeting and hanging out with the other girls. I kept it all bottled up inside.

I also never discussed the terror I felt when I learned that, after physical education at school, all the girls were required to take a shower together. That meant I'd have to be naked in front of everyone. The idea freaked me out. I thought of not showering at all, but the teachers carefully checked to make sure we did what we were told.

The godsend was a single-stall shower off by itself, with a curtain for privacy. I'm not sure we were supposed to use it, but I didn't care. When it was time to shower, I ran like hell to that isolated shower and claimed it as my own. I was able to avoid exposing what I perceived to be my flawed and flabby body.

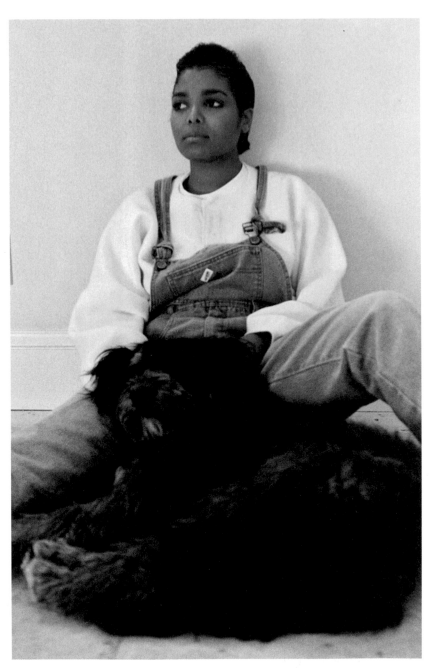

With Puffy. I loved her to pieces. This dog was my life. Even though I feel she is in heaven, our souls are still connected. I miss her still. We shared a true love. Puffy was always family to me. Puffy's love was unconditional.

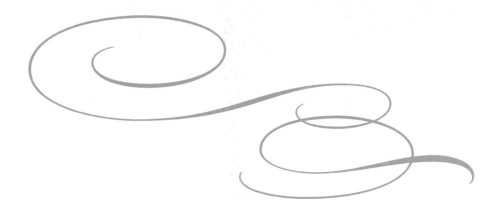

God and Dogs

My childhood was a powerful and often perplexing combination of experiences that were wonderful as well as challenging. One of the more challenging experiences happened when I was nine and attending public school.

It began harmlessly. The teacher said she was looking for a

student to solve a simple math problem. First the student would go stand in front of the classroom. Then the teacher would ask the question. Were there any volunteers? No hands went up.

"I guess I'll have to call on someone," the teacher said.

I prayed that she wouldn't call on me.

But she did.

My heart started hammering. I was good at math, but suddenly all confidence left me. As I walked to the front of the class, I was assaulted with negative thoughts—*What if I don't understand her question? What if I don't know the answer? What if I make a fool of myself?*

When the question was asked, my mind was too riddled with doubts to even hear it clearly. I asked the teacher to repeat the problem.

But hearing it again made no difference. My head was filled with confusion. I panicked. I couldn't speak; I just stood there.

"Janet," the teacher said, "this couldn't be easier. You have to know the answer."

That only made things worse. As I stood there speechless, other kids started throwing their hands up in the air, begging to be chosen. They were practically groaning—that's how eager they were to scream out the answer. I felt dumb. I wanted to die. I wanted to run out of the room and keep running forever.

That incident has stayed with me. I've rewound the tape in my mind and watched it over and over again. I've dreamed about it and, decades after it happened, have talked about it. Now I'm writing about it. I realize today how much it affected me when I had to do public speaking: I hated such situations because they always reminded me of that schoolroom trauma, which had deepened my shyness and fear of facing a group of strangers. If I'm onstage, I'm fine. Being onstage is like being at home. I've grown up onstage. But if the stage is a classroom or a press conference, I'm unhappy and reluctant to say much of anything. That small move from my seat to a position in front of the class changed my life. I felt as though I was unfairly labeled incompetent or, even worse, stupid.

"It felt like I was being condemned for something beyond my control," said my friend whose stutter kept him from the junior debate team when he was ten. "I was already an advanced reader. And I could argue as well as anyone. But because I had trouble getting the words out, I was told that wasn't acceptable."

Fortunately, that didn't stop him. A casting director from a theater company was recruiting for kids' roles in grown-up plays. My friend auditioned and was selected.

"Something wonderful happened when I started acting," he said. "I could lose myself in another character and suddenly my stutter was gone. I was especially good at playing characters who were scared. I used my own fears about speaking to understand their fears—and somehow my own speaking was transformed."

I related. I felt closest to the true me when I was presented with the challenge of acting.

When I acted onstage during those early skits, some saw me as a little doll. But I didn't see myself that way. I was an actress playing a part. Yet I also *was* a young girl, who looked at dolls as objects to adore. Dolls were beautiful. Dolls were the perfect shape.

Dolls could not get too thin or too fat. Like me, dolls were quiet. Dolls were too shy to talk. They just stared at you lovingly. I also saw dolls in love with one another.

I'd have the girl dolls and boy dolls sleep in one another's arms. And before I had any understanding of sex, I would undress the dolls and arrange their bodies so that they embraced. I did it because it seemed that, in their most natural state, they were the most loving. The dolls were not anatomically accurate, and I wasn't thinking about anything lewd. I was just thinking about couples who, unlike my own parents, could express a close and tender relationship.

The doll I wanted most was Malibu Barbie. She had hair down to her waist and a one-piece aqua bathing suit. Naturally, she wore sunglasses and carried a yellow towel and a bottle of suntan lotion. There was a pop-up beach tent for Barbie's naps, in addition to a dream house complete with elevator and swimming pool. I wanted the whole package, and I wanted it badly. If there were any black dolls of any kind, they didn't have their own commercials or beach houses like Malibu Barbie did.

Mother said no. Mother often said no. And looking back, I'm grateful that we Jacksons did not get everything we wanted. Our parents were careful about not indulging us. Our childhood was about serious work.

We lived on an estate that covered three acres, but that only meant we kids had to do our part to take care of it all. Mike, Randy, and I raked leaves every Saturday morning. My sister La Toya mopped the floors to perfection, never leaving a single smudge. Jermaine vacuumed. We fed and bathed our animals. In the case of some of the more exotic animals, we bottle-fed them when they were small. We cleaned their cages and kept them groomed.

Inside the house, Mike, Randy, and I cleaned the windows with newspapers—no streaks allowed. When we washed dishes, we used scalding hot water. We made our own beds. We didn't mind these tasks and, in fact, sang to one another as we worked. When I was asked to do something alone—carry the trash out to the end of the driveway, for example—I'd use the opportunity to speak to God. I would confide my fears and feelings of inadequacy. I realize now that that was the beginning of my spiritual journey.

When I was down—say, after a difficult day at school—I'd talk to my dogs, Black Girl, Lobo, and Heavy. I told them my innermost feelings, and I felt like they understood. I felt safe in doing so because a dog's love is one thing you can count on. Your dog doesn't judge you. In many ways, like God, dogs *are* love.

It was always difficult talking to my father, who made us call him Joseph, not Dad. He was a man of action, not words. And the truth is that we feared him. I was the last of nine children, and I believe that by the time I was born my parents had grown tired of disciplining. They were more lenient with me and Randy, the next to youngest, than with our older siblings. There was one time, however, when my father hit me.

I can't remember what rule I had disobeyed, but I had just stepped out of the bathtub when he struck me with his belt. It left marks on my skin. It's interesting that I don't recall the lesson my father was trying to teach, only the violence he used to make his point. Violence has a way of overwhelming everything. I think my father is misunderstood. It's important for you to know that my father loves all of his children and that his way of communicating his love was a result of his upbringing. I tell this story not to judge him, but to be open and to break the cycle.

Fear can also be overwhelming. Many nights my siblings and I would put on our pajamas and go to Mother's room. We would tell jokes, read stories, and watch TV. We felt safe there. In between our laughter, we'd sometimes hear the crunching sound of tires rolling up the gravel driveway. It was Joseph in his car, headlights turned off, windows rolled down, trying to sneak up on us to hear what we were talking about. The sound of his car stopped us cold. We'd scatter like roaches, off to our rooms, ducking down low so not to be visible through the windows. We didn't know what mood Joseph was bringing home.

I know that my kind of story is not uncommon, and I know many have endured far worse. Through it all we always had Mother's love as a constant, and so many people don't even have that. But it is important to remember that with an unstable foundation, you can't find your own true you.

I'm certain I received less of his wrath than my other siblings did, but there were times when Joseph began screaming at me for reasons I didn't comprehend. I now understand that he has an issue with anger management. My father's love for us, his passion for us to succeed, his burning desire to provide for his children, were sometimes communicated in anger. I wish I had understood then what I understand today. But as children, when we face anger— anger that strikes us unexpectedly, like a lightning bolt—we have no real protection. We presume either that we did wrong or simply *are* wrong, through and through.

Before Joseph initiated my professional career apart from the family, Mother put me in ballet class when I was six. She had good motives. I would learn posture, movement, and grace. But unfortunately, I was bored to death. I hated wearing leotards. Then one day the teacher struck me, claiming that I was ignoring her directions to tuck in my booty.

"I'm trying," I said, and I was. She didn't think I was trying hard enough. I thought it was the very size of my booty that bothered her—because there was simply no way I could tuck it any further. In any event, she lost her temper, hit me, and left me embarrassed and hurt. Mother learned what had happened and never made me return.

When I was a teen, Mother suggested I give ballet another chance, this time with a private male instructor. At the end of a lesson, he put his hands on my face and got extremely close to me. I thought he was going to kiss me, and I turned away. It was creepy. I told Mother, who stopped the lessons right then and there.

Mother, bless her heart, was always trying to make a lady of me. At the same time she was fiercely protective. Joseph, on the hand, was more interested in activating my career. If it weren't for him, I would never have received national attention for something I did on my own.

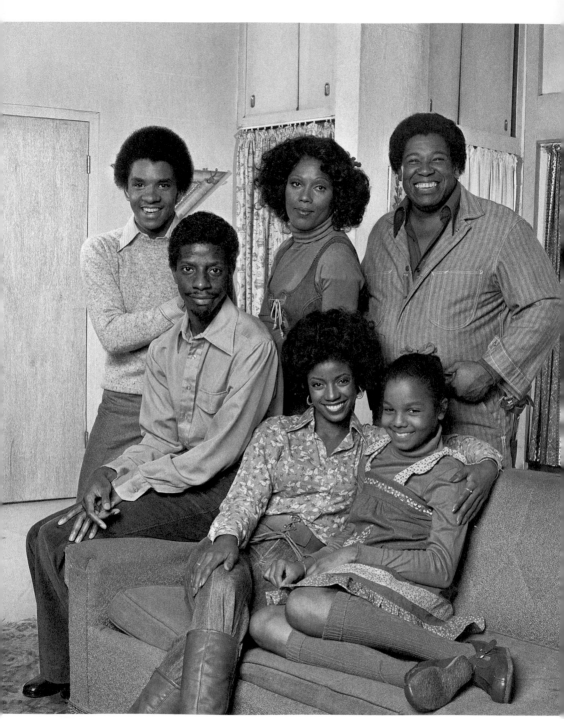

On the set of *Good Times*.

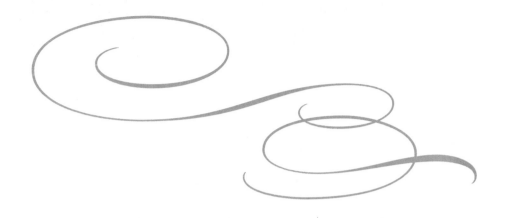

Good Times

My acting career began on a serious note when my father got a call from the office of television producer Norman Lear, inquiring about my availability for a situation comedy.

In the mid-1970s, Norman Lear was the king of television. He had created *All in the Family* and *Maude*, among other shows.

Good Times was a spin-off from *Maude* and at this point, 1977, was starring Ja'Net DuBois. Lear was looking for a young girl to play Ja'Net's foster child, Penny. According to the script, the child had endured physical abuse at the hands of her biological mother.

I knew none of this when Mother and I arrived at the production office. I didn't know who Lear was, and I didn't understand how significant it was that he himself was conducting the audition.

Lear began by chatting amiably with me. I sensed that he was a nice man. Then he asked me a question that threw me.

"Janet," he said, "are you able to cry?"

I thought that was a strange question.

"Everyone can cry, Mr. Lear," I said.

"But can you cry on cue, Janet? Can you cry when I ask you to?"

"I'm not sure," I answered honestly.

"Let me give you an example," he said. "Let's say you bought me a gift, a beautiful blue tie, that you think is perfect for me. You're absolutely convinced that this gift will thrill me. You've picked it out because it matches my eyes. You can't wait to give to me. Okay?"

"Okay," I said.

"Now," Lear continued, "hand me this tie. Go ahead and hand it to me."

I handed him an invisible tie.

He responded by saying, "How could you give me such an ugly tie? I don't like it."

Right then and there, tears slowly started to run down my face.

"But I bought it for you," I said. "It matches your eyes."

"I don't want it."

My tears kept flowing. I felt genuinely hurt. I couldn't hold back my true feelings.

"Good," Lear said, now smiling. "Very good."

I wiped my eyes.

"That will be all, Janet," he said. "We'll be in touch with you."

I knew how auditions worked—you either got a callback or not. I normally presumed the worst.

Mother and I got up and left the room. When we reached the hallway, she kissed me on the cheek and said, "You did fine, baby."

"Do you think I can have Malibu Barbie now?" I asked.

"Not yet," Mother said.

Before we left the building, though, Lear called us back. When we reentered the office, he sat us down and said it simply. "Janet was so good we've decided to call off the other auditions. Your daughter has the part. Congratulations."

"What do you say about that, Janet?" Mother said.

"Thank you, Mr. Lear," I said.

I felt happy all over, but I also felt moved to ask Mother the question all over again. "Do you think I can have Malibu Barbie now?"

"Yes, baby," she said. And from Lear's Tandem Productions office we made a beeline to Toys 'R' Us, where I raced down the aisle and grabbed the whole package—the tent, the pool, the dream house, and, of course, Miss Barbie herself.

It's ironic that while I was buying a Barbie dream house, the character that I was cast to play in *Good Times,* Penny, was living a nightmare. She was going through horrible times. She was an abused and beaten child who suffered terribly at the hands of her mother. Her mother burned her with an iron and broke her arm. I was asked to play someone who, although smiling and sweet on the outside, had an interior life of extreme fear and pain.

To help me through the process, I leaned on my real-life siblings. On those first shows, I wore Randy's jeans because they fit me better than my own. La Toya helped me learn my lines, and so did my Mike, who was just about to go off to New York and film *The Wiz.* During rehearsals, I wouldn't cry. I don't know why. I just blocked the feelings. Maybe they were too much for me. When it came time to tape, though, the tears flowed. I felt what I needed to feel. I felt how much Penny needed to be loved.

I felt love from the cast of *Good Times,* who became a second family to me. However, I was still uncomfortable with the process. I hated the table readings. That's when we were asked to read the scripts out loud. I didn't think of myself as a good reader. I'd stumble over words. I'd feel everyone's eyes focused on me.

I was also told that I was overweight and immediately needed to slim down. In the very first episode, the wardrobe department told me they had to bind my breasts. Where the decision came from, I will never know. So now it was not just my butt; it was my chest, too. I was in constant discomfort and lacked self-assurance.

The other young actresses that I knew in passing appeared to be self-composed. At the studio next to ours, two girls—Valerie Bertinelli and Mackenzie Phillips—were doing *One Day at a Time*. They seemed to know what they were doing. I wasn't sure that I did. Today I understand that Valerie and Mackenzie were fighting battles of their own.

But I did it anyway. I acted. I pretended. I kept up a grinding work schedule. I missed my family like crazy—Mike, who was making *The Wiz;* my other siblings, who were always recording. Meanwhile, I was working on this TV show nine to five.

Nonetheless, I was grateful for the part and the opportunity to act. I also derived satisfaction out of being on time and doing my work. My mom was supportive and loving. My brothers, whom I had once watched as cartoon characters on TV, said that they now liked watching me.

As a result of my success on *Good Times,* I was beginning to develop a small amount of self-esteem. I had accomplished something on my own, apart from my family. I had proven that I could act. The problem, though, is that the self-esteem was overwhelmed by self-doubt. I still did not see myself as attractive or especially talented. I figured I had gotten a lucky break. Because acting at the beginning didn't seem especially difficult, I couldn't give myself much credit for being good at it. In fact, I could hardly give myself credit for anything.

Yes, I was disciplined. Yes, I was being recognized. Yes, I was operating in the difficult realm of show business. But deep inside, did I feel uniquely blessed? Did I feel truly worthy?

The feeling that comes when you know the true you—a

true you that is strong, sincere, beautiful, and unquestionably valuable—was a long ways off. Before I could embrace that feeling, there was a world of lessons to be learned. And maybe because I see myself as a slow learner, none of the lessons were easy.

Yes, I was disciplined. Yes, I was being recognized. Yes, I was operating in the difficult realm of show business. But deep inside did I feel uniquely blessed? Did I feel truly worthy?

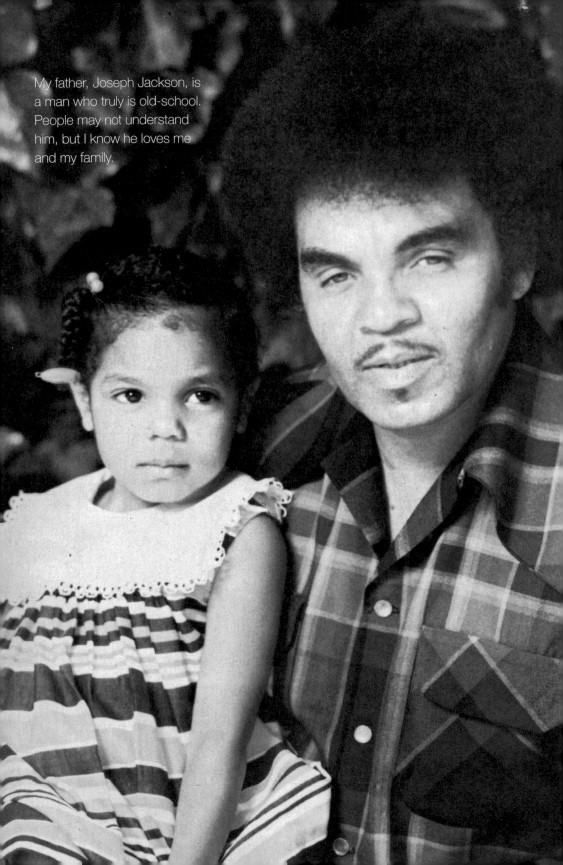

My father, Joseph Jackson, is a man who truly is old-school. People may not understand him, but I know he loves me and my family.

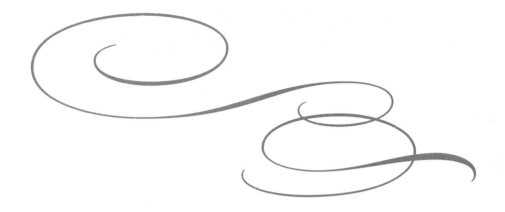

Discipline

Our family was all about discipline. My parents saw discipline as the key to survival and success. I never once rebelled against the notion of hard work, practice, and rigorous rehearsal. I didn't always like it—after all, I was a kid—but watching my brothers do it and seeing the results, the message was clear: no discipline, no achievement.

When it came time to get up in the morning and head to the set of *Good Times,* I was out of bed before the alarm clock rang. I was dressed. I was prompt. I was programmed. I embraced my family's sense of unyielding discipline. I am the product of that discipline and cannot envision my life without it.

And yet . . .

When it came to food, the concept of discipline didn't exist. I was given no instructions about what or when to eat. We were a show business family focused on show business success. Food was fuel to keep us going. Food was necessary, but hardly required study.

In the early days, when I went on the road with my brothers, it was all about room service. In fact, it became a running joke that little Janet had memorized the room service numbers at every hotel on the circuit. I loved calling up and ordering whatever I liked—cheeseburgers, or apple pie, whatever and whenever. It was magical. Pick up the phone, and thirty minutes later there it was: my fondest desire arrived on a silver platter.

Disciplined artistic training came to me as naturally as eating, yet when it came to eating, discipline flew out the window.

Some of my siblings, such as my sister La Toya, have high metabolisms. La Toya could eat dozens of her beloved chocolate turtles without gaining a pound.

My metabolism was slow.

My appetite was big.

After a show, after receiving a standing ovation, I wanted to celebrate the good feeling. I would go back to the hotel room and make a phone call.

The waiter would wheel in the food—hamburgers, french fries, and ice cream.

If someone had told me back then that just as I needed to be a disciplined actor, I also needed to be a disciplined eater, I wouldn't have understood. Though I was hardly a rebellious kid, I would have surely rejected the idea of curbing my eating habits.

Eating was emotional for me; eating calmed my nerves and brought me instant gratification.

"I hated the word *discipline*," a friend of mine once told me. "My mother was a rabid disciplinarian. If I got out of bed a minute late, I was punished. If I didn't eat every last bite of my oatmeal, I was punished. If my homework wasn't finished by eight, even more punishment. As a result, I was always late getting out of bed, I never finished my oatmeal, and I never completed my homework on time. I flat-out rebelled. I couldn't stand the pressure, and I resented how everything had to be just so.

" 'Why?' I asked my mother. 'Why can't I stay in bed another five minutes? Why can't I have another hour to get through with my homework?'

" 'Because you need to learn discipline' was always her answer.

" 'What's the big deal about discipline?' I wanted to know.

" 'Without discipline, you'll never amount to anything.'

"Well, when you're seven or eight years old, the idea of 'amounting to something' isn't foremost on your mind, is it?"

"But at least it showed you that your mother cared," I said.

"I didn't feel that she cared about me," my friend said. "I felt like she cared about this principle of discipline. Discipline was just making me do things I didn't want to do when I didn't want to do them. Her insistence on discipline turned me into a wild child."

For all the truth in my friend's story, I saw the positive side of discipline. I didn't reject or resist discipline, because I saw how discipline led to success. Success meant pleasing an audience and earning a standing ovation.

I was still a preteen when Mike introduced us to vegetarianism. I believe that came out of his love for animals, a love that I share deeply. It seemed to make sense, and the majority of the family went along with the program. Mother agreed and felt it was not only important to exclude animal flesh from our diet but to employ colonic treatments on a weekly basis. The idea was that the bacteria and toxins that accumulate in the colon have to be flushed out. Later I would learn that many doctors disagree with this method, feeling that the body's digestive system naturally eliminates those toxins. There is a school of thought, however, that maintaining a healthy colon requires extraordinary measures. For many years, our family adopted those measures. And as an obedient child, I didn't argue or challenge the plan. As a young girl, that wasn't my nature.

Because I loved Mike and cherished the times he and I spent together, I was more than willing to embrace his diet. That became another bond between us. Before he recorded *Off the Wall*, he could go out in public without security. People recognized him and asked for autographs, but it was still manageable and not intrusive. We'd go out alone.

He'd drive us from the San Fernando Valley to a vegetarian restaurant run by Sikhs on Third Street in Los Angeles, called the Golden Temple. We'd eat salads and drink Yogi tea. The meals were delicious, and we stuffed ourselves. I remember thinking—or hoping—that overeating healthy food wouldn't get me fat the way nonhealthy food might. I still worried, however, that healthy or not, I was too fat and that my eating was out of control. But these were private worries; I didn't mention them to Mike. At the same time, Mike, who had problems with acne, never discussed that with me. All of us in our family—brothers, sisters, mother, and father— kept such thoughts to ourselves.

There were also wonderful spontaneous trips that Mike and I would make to give food to the homeless. We'd buy a bunch of takeout meals and drive around the city, stopping whenever we saw someone holding a sign asking for help. That was Mike's idea of a good time—simply give to the poor on a personal basis. All this happened when I was still a preteen and Mike was not yet twenty. Our closeness meant the world to me. There was still taunting about my booty or my inability to trim down, but that was more than compensated by our private time together. I saw no problems on the horizon.

"I did," said my sister La Toya years later. "I always knew you'd have weight issues."

"Why?" I asked.

"The teasing got to you. I saw it in your face. You might have said, 'Sticks and stones might hurt my bones, but names will never harm me,' but I knew that the names were harming you."

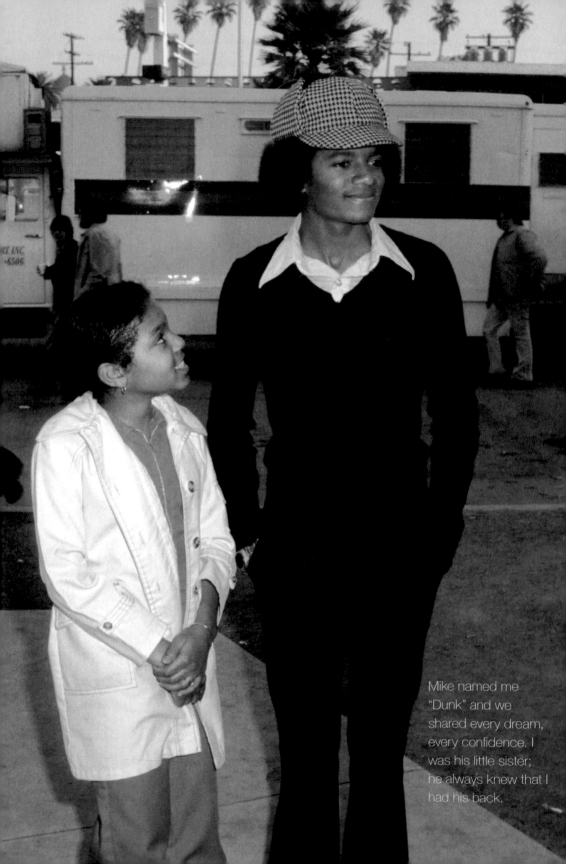

Mike named me
"Dunk" and we
shared every dream,
every confidence. I
was his little sister;
he always knew that I
had his back.

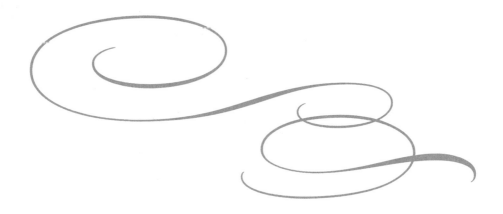

Escapade

I was eleven and on break from *Good Times* when Mike invited me to New York. It was 1977, and the height of disco madness. La Toya was also there. Excitedly, Mike told me about this club called Studio 54. Nightclubs weren't anything new for me. My siblings had been taking me to clubs for years. I was used to being the only kid at the party. But from the minute we arrived, I knew this was different.

Long lines of people, dressed in fabulous outfits, were waiting to get in. Once we were spotted, we were whisked right inside. The place was mammoth. It was packed. Strobe lights flashing. People sniffing flour.

"Why are they doing that?" I asked, not understanding that it wasn't flour they were sniffing. No one answered me. Everyone was too busy looking.

I was introduced to the owners, Steve Rubell and Ian Schrager. I saw Liza Minnelli. I recognized her from her films and knew that her mother was Judy Garland. I also knew the films of her father, Vincente Minnelli. I also recognized the man she was with— Halston. It was a dazzling, amazing scene. I don't think I said a single word the entire night.

I felt privileged to be there. With the exception of Brooke Shields, what other young kid could gain entrance? It was a fascinating glimpse into the world of extreme celebrity glamour.

Mike could have excluded me from such experiences. But in his mind—and in mine—such experiences were fun. It was plain fun to see the outlandishness of one of the wildest clubs ever to host the stars.

To be included was to be loved.

I cherish such experiences. Despite whatever self-image issues I had—feeling I was fat, or a poor student, or inferior to my siblings—the presence of my family was and remains a comfort. Families can be challenging, and many are deeply dysfunctional.

But despite that dysfunction, a family can provide a loving energy that's hard, if not impossible, to duplicate.

Long ago a friend told me this story that I'll never forget. It's testimony to the strength of family, even when that family comprises just two people.

"When I was a little girl," she said, "I lived alone with my father. My mom had died in childbirth and all four of his grandparents lived far away. It was just Daddy and me. Daddy had problems. He was a drinker, and he couldn't hold down a job. We were always moving the day before the rent was due. I changed elementary school five or six times. Usually I was the one who had to wake up Daddy so he could take me to school. I was very young—five or six—when I started making him breakfast. I didn't know the word for it then, but I do now: he was depressed. It was hard for him to get out of bed and get going. In the evenings, we ate frozen dinners or takeout from McDonald's. When I got older, Daddy wasn't really capable of helping me with my homework.

"Once in a while he'd have a lady friend help me. One of his girlfriends was a bookkeeper and good at math. Another worked at the library and helped me with my reading. But Daddy wasn't good at keeping these relationships. He'd quickly move from one lady to another. I often heard him fighting with them over the phone or in person. He had all sorts of problems that I could talk about for days, or years, or even the rest of my life.

"But here's what I remember most, and here's what I cling to most—the fact that my father was there. Every night when I went to sleep, he was there. Every morning when I awoke, he was there. I know that he fed me the wrong foods and I know that he never had the right stuff to fight the demons that kept him down. But the simple fact that he stuck around—day in and day out—told me the one thing I needed to know. That he cared. And because he cared, I was able to feel that I was worth caring for."

Being in the real world
taught me that when it
comes to relationships,
it is all about sincerity,
not class, or race, or
economic status.

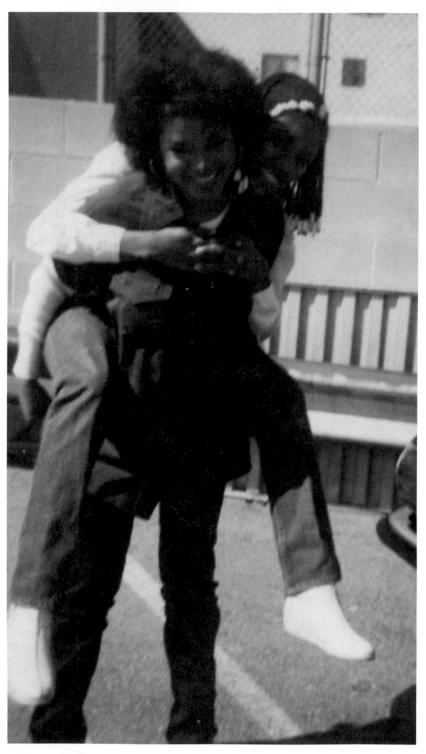

With my childhood friend La Nette. In high school, feeling fat even though I was so thin.

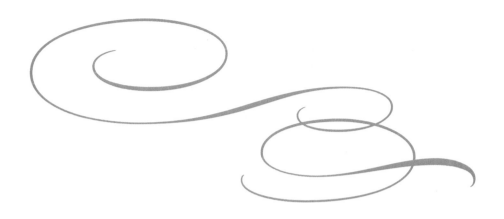

All Right

At the end of my stint on *Good Times*, I had to enroll in a new school. I no longer needed to be tutored privately. I had to go to a real school with real kids and deal with my real issues. It was one of the biggest changes in my young life up to this point. I was nervous and not happy. I was struggling with how I looked and whether I would fit in with the new kids. I would be out of my comfort zone.

New school, new kids, and new teachers. I would be without Mrs. Fine, the wonderful woman who had privately tutored me and my brothers. I couldn't imagine any teachers would be as nice or patient as her. She came with us on the road. She was there when I did *Good Times*. Mrs. Fine was an angel, my second mother. And she always told me, Randy, and Mike that we were her children from another lifetime.

When I wasn't being tutored, I had had Mrs. Womack—my fourth-grade teacher and the only black teacher I ever had. She was a sweet and reassuring presence in the classroom. Now she wouldn't be there to watch over me, to reassure me.

If I could have, at age twelve I would have wound back the clock to the time when I had school with my siblings in hotel suites. But those times were gone.

I would have to go to school and be normal. I would have to somehow fit in.

The first day in this new school put me in a guarded and negative mood. Yet within minutes, my mood magically changed. Something happened that I hadn't dreamed possible. Busloads of black and Latin kids were arriving from south-central Los Angeles to attend this school in the Valley.

These kids would change my outlook on life.

It wasn't that I had anything against the white kids. I had grown up in a white environment and when I was in school, my classmates and teachers were white. Those kids were (and some remain) very close friends.

But something happened inside my heart when I saw black and Latin kids my age stepping off that bus. I was excited to see them.

That good feeling spread during lunchtime. There, outside in the yard, the black kids congregated in one area around a boom box blasting Funkadelic's "One Nation Under a Groove." When they started dancing, the sight of them moving with such smooth style and funky grace thrilled me.

A girl named La Nette, who lived in the Crenshaw district of Los Angeles, a world away from the Valley, became my best friend.

She knew I was a Jackson—everyone did—and said she had seen me on *Good Times,* but she wasn't starstruck in the least. She treated me the same way she treated her other friends, with natural ease and friendliness. When she invited me to her house one weekend, I asked Mother if she'd drive me over.

"Of course, baby," she said.

And she did.

As Mother navigated the freeways to Crenshaw, I was excited by a new friendship in a new part of the city where normal black folks lived. Mother turned up the volume on her favorite Kenny Rogers tape. Mother was a country music fan. The music made the long trip seem short.

When I arrived at La Nette's house, we hung out and she played me her favorites—George Clinton & Parliament's "Knee Deep," Foxy's "Get Off," and Teena Marie and Rick James's "Fire & Desire." It was a beautiful exchange, the songs that she loved and the ones I loved. It was even more beautiful to be part of the real world. To fit in. To be all right not just with these kids but with myself.

My first day at school was different from everyone else's, because of the *Good Times* schedule. There were moments when my presence was distracting to the entire class because of the work I was doing in TV, and because of my family. I can remember being sent to the principal's office just to have a quiet place to do my schoolwork when things got crazy. Growing up, I'd seen others in similar situations, but I didn't realize how strange it was until I was an adult. It was a lesson in being different.

In this world, I wasn't a Jackson. I was just Janet. And that was enough.

Being in the real world taught me that when it comes to relationships, it's all about sincerity, not class, or race, or economic status. I found that I was comfortable with straightforward, genuine people. I could relate to them and they could relate to me. I found myself comfortable in any world whose people had open hearts.

That was a valuable lesson I'll carry for the rest of my life. Sincerity sees you through any situation.

Another extracurricular lesson these kids taught me was humility. Seeing how I was privileged—and how many of my new friends were not—humbled me. Their firsthand stories of life in the inner city were powerful and moving. They experienced great joy and great pain. I loved these kids. We were one, and we were together. We were never against the other students at school, yet we formed a special bond among ourselves.

By my final months at school, though, there was racial tension. Later in my life, this awakening would reemerge in the sounds and stories of *Rhythm Nation*.

Perhaps my own lack
of self-respect had me
believing that I wasn't
worthy of a relationship in
which, besides addressing
the needs of someone
else, I could have my
own needs met.

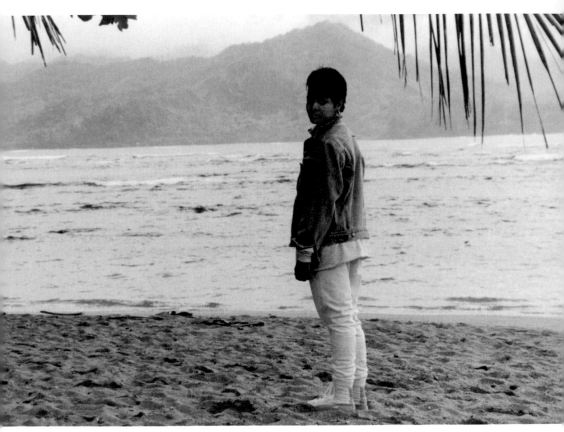

On the beach in Hawaii. Just turned twenty-one. Moments before, I was proposed to. I didn't know the engagement was coming or what would follow.

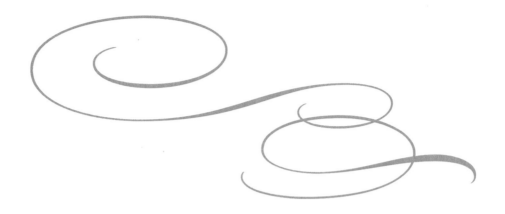

"Young Love"

I was sixteen when I gave my virginity to my first love, James De-Barge. My general reaction: "This is it? This is what everyone has been talking about?"

It was awkward and painful. Eventually the pain went away, but for a long time lovemaking was far from a thrilling experience.

James later became my husband. He was nineteen, a sweet and loving young man. He was more experienced sexually than me, and I certainly don't blame him for the initial difficulties I had enjoying physical intimacy. We loved each other, and I was sure that I wanted to be with him for the rest of my life.

I was wrong. James was a good guy with major faults. I was convinced that I could fix him, but I didn't know that "fixing" wasn't my job. And even if it had been my job, I didn't know how to do it. I didn't realize the seriousness of the challenges he faced. I didn't have any idea about his many internal conflicts—and how deep they were. Finally, as a teenager, I simply couldn't fathom the complexities of love.

In *Romeo and Juliet,* a tragedy some call the best play about romance ever written, Juliet is thirteen. Shakespeare doesn't give Romeo's age, although he's likely also a teenager. Yet their love is profound, and embodies a sweet spirituality that has captured the hearts and imaginations of readers for more than four hundred years.

Isn't teen love real?

It sure has its own kind of reality.

I know that in my own case I was involved on a very deep emotional level. I loved and cared for James with all my heart. When he was in trouble, I was there for him. I wanted to help him, and wanted to save him from himself. It was a long period of anguish for me. Night after night, I cried my eyes out. I wanted it to work, but it never would.

We had both been raised in show business families. We could relate—or least we thought we could. James faced tremendous emotional challenges with drug addiction. For reasons I don't entirely understand even to this day, I took on the role of caretaker. When he was down, it was my job to lift him up. When he disappeared, I had to go find him. I had to keep him from destroying himself.

I can only guess why I put myself in such a thankless position. Perhaps my own lack of self-respect had me believing that I wasn't worthy of a relationship in which, besides addressing the needs of someone else, I could have my own needs met.

Confusing matters even more was our position in the world of entertainment. We were entertainers; our siblings were entertainers; our parents were involved in our careers; we lived in the spotlight; and we were both overstimulated by the demands and insecurities of the business. We really didn't have a chance.

I recently heard from a woman I'll call Sonya.

"I was in love at thirteen," she said. "I know it was love. I'm not saying it was mature love or adult love, but what difference does that make? It was its own kind of love. The feelings in my heart were so powerful that *love* is the only word strong enough to describe it. All I could do was think about this boy. I had to be with him every minute of the day. I'd write his name in my notebook a hundred times over. I'd call him ten times a day. He was three years older than me. He was cute and smart. He had a soft, sexy voice and beautiful hands. He liked me because I liked *him* so much. I flattered him with my crazy attention. I'd write these love letters that went on for pages and pages. I knew he showed them to his friends as something of a joke, but I didn't care. As long as he took me out.

"Of course, I was going to have sex with him. That wasn't even a question. He could have whatever he wanted from me. The sex, though, was not very good. I didn't know how, and neither did he. So we just fumbled around and barely managed to connect. He made me promise that I wouldn't tell anyone that he was awkward, and I agreed. But naturally he went around bragging about everything he'd done with me. He told his friends that I was a freak. Even that, though, didn't bother me. As long as he kept me by his side.

"My parents saw what was happening and said I was sick. They sent me to a shrink who said the same thing. She was this uptight woman who threw around words like *compulsive* and *obsessive* and recommended that I see her two times a week. But I only wanted to see my boyfriend. I refused help because I didn't think I needed any. All I needed was him.

"Finally we figured out the lovemaking thing. It was never great but good enough to get me pregnant. I had turned fourteen. My mother was against an abortion, and so was I. I was sent to live with an aunt in another state and have my baby there. My boyfriend couldn't have cared less. 'I'm not even your boyfriend,' he said. 'I don't care what you do.'

"I moved to my aunt's, where I continued calling him every day. By now, though, he refused to talk to me. I did nothing but cry night and day, and only stopped when I had a miscarriage. That lifeless fetus became a symbol of my lifeless love. My deep, deep depression lasted for the rest of junior high and high school. I never had another boyfriend till college. And even then, the relationship was short-lived. I couldn't trust a man with my heart.

"When I look back, I see that the very thing I didn't have was the thing I needed most—someone to talk to. That someone couldn't be my mother because she wasn't ready to listen to me, especially about things like love and sex. That someone couldn't be the therapist because she was cold and distant. My father was even more distant and, an only child, I had practically no female friends. I needed to talk to other girls who were going through what I was going through—heavy-duty teen love. I needed to hear how other girls were not only willing but eager to lose themselves, as I had lost myself, in some guy that they had turned into a god.

"Again, I'm not saying it wasn't love. It was love. And the more my parents or anyone said I was too young to be in love, the less I listened to them. Teen love is love. But teen love is a crazy love. It was the only kind of love I was able to express at that time. The problem, though, was I had nowhere to go to talk about this love—and no one capable of opening their heart to what I had to say."

Sonya's story brings up so many issues. The main one, though, is how she undervalued herself. I related. I remembered.

Teens have tremendous pressure on them.

Parents are overprotective or not protective enough.

Sex is a constant challenge.

Body image is always there. Body parts growing too fast or not fast enough. Skin problems. Hair problems. Too heavy, too thin, too wide, too narrow.

The technological toys are delights and distractions at the same time. Everyone is texting, tweeting, messaging, surfing. Everyone is multitasking to the point that attention spans are reduced to nothing. Four seconds for this task. Two seconds for that one. Click on, click off.

Who can think?

Who can reflect?

Who can stop and say, "Hey, it's time just to listen to my breath and realize I'm alive"?

If teens were confused before—and God knows, I was—the confusion is tenfold these days.

I was a confused teenager without being told that it was not only okay to be confused, but in fact perfectly natural.

I try to imagine what it would have felt like to hear those simple words spoken directly to me:

Janet, it's okay to be confused. Confusion is normal. If you're confused, there's nothing wrong with you. You can live with confusion. Confusion is part of growing up.

To be given permission to be confused—and remain confused—for as long as it takes would have been a huge gift.

What's wrong with confusion if confusion is real?

To cut off the confusion and accept an answer just because it's too scary not to have an answer is a good way to get the wrong answer.

Living with confusion is part of life.

Embracing confusion is a courageous and honest way to live.

Admitting confusion is the quickest way to move past confusion.

I'm often confused—about professional choices, or private choices. I don't like to announce that fact. But if I admit it to close friends or associates, I find myself more relaxed. I've admitted the truth. Now let me slowly work my way out of the confusion by weighing all the alternatives, thinking clearly, and reaching a reasonable conclusion.

I guess it all goes back to the strength we gain from exposing our vulnerability. Don't get me wrong. I love being certain. I love being absolutely sure about a course of action. But if the certainty isn't there, it isn't there, and I have to deal with doubt. To deny doubt—to cover it up—is to deny your reality. And that makes matters even worse.

It's taken me a lifetime to learn, and to admit, that it's okay to be confused.

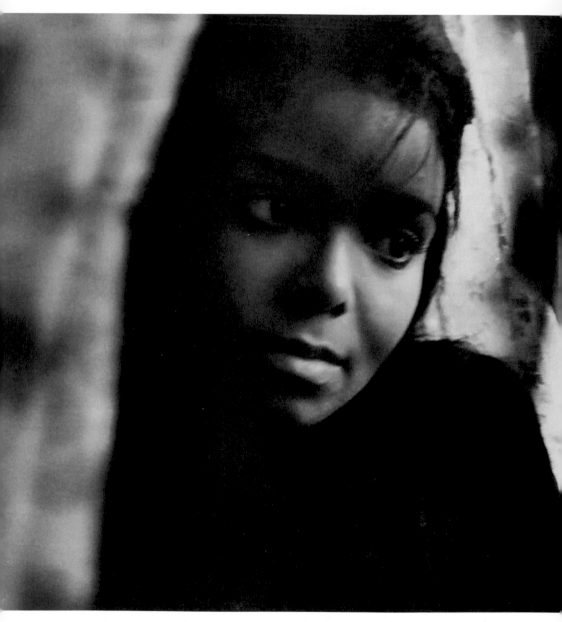

Living back at home—briefly with my parents—after my first marriage
ended.

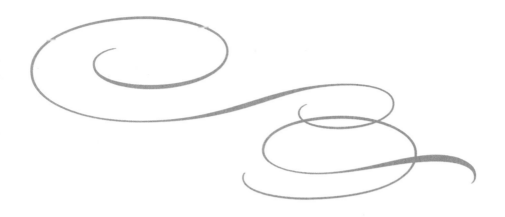

Fame

While James and I were together, I was cast on *Fame*. Though I loved acting and wanted to pursue it, I wasn't excited about this television show, and if it had been left up to me, I would have passed. Joseph, though, insisted that I take the role of Cleo Hewitt—so, still the obedient child, I acquiesced. The experience was trying.

I was taking birth control bills and as a result, I ballooned so much that people on the show thought I was pregnant. Once again, producers were telling me that I looked too big, that I needed to be thinner, and that I was presenting the wrong image to the public. These years, roughly from the ages of sixteen to eighteen, were not happy ones for me. The kids on *Fame* were not treated well. We had to use public bathrooms in the studio and were given ill-equipped dressing rooms that were so tiny we could barely change in them.

Some of the cast members were real jokesters. I'd often open my breakfast case and find the food missing. Someone would take it just to tease me. The kids would blow pot smoke into my dressing room, knowing that smoke gave me a terrible headache. They were already a family. It was like an initiation, a rite of passage, and I was the new kid on the block.

In my heart, all I wanted to do was work out my relationship with James. But how? I'd be out until 2 A.M., looking for him on the streets. Then I'd have to get up at four to be at the set by six. I was often late. I think I wanted to get fired. Fortunately, they did let me go. I had a three-year contract but was released after the first year. Meanwhile, my relationship with James was collapsing, and our brief marriage was annulled.

I was feeling belittled even while I was still feeling fat. The result was more emotional eating—eating to chase away the blues, eating to beat back fears.

What were my fears?

That I would never find love that would last, that I would

repeat the failure of my marriage, or that I would remain forever fat? I'm not sure.

It was touching to see that other young women my age also had a troublesome relationship with their body image. Around this time, I received a long letter from someone I'll call Sheila, a teenager who had a story much different from mine. Yet I related deeply.

Sheila was reed-thin, and up until she was fifteen, she had never had problems with weight. On the contrary, her brothers called her a scarecrow and her mother was always saying that she was emaciated. In response, Sheila said that she wanted to be a model and liked her body just the way it was.

She wasn't ready to have sex with her boyfriend. When he insisted, she still resisted. That's when he forced her. Now they call it date rape, but back then Sheila didn't have a name for what happened. Shocked, confused, and afraid, she locked the secret inside her heart. Twelve months later, she had gained nearly seventy pounds. Her family didn't know what to think.

"You've turned from scarecrow to pig," said her brother.

"It's one thing to gain a little weight," her mom said, "but you look absolutely grotesque."

Despite her attempt to curb her eating, she couldn't. She became obsessed with food, especially breads and sweets. The doctor put her on a program, which she ignored. She kept getting heavier. It was only when a teacher at school suggested that she see a psychologist, a suggestion her mother called ridiculous, that Sheila experienced a breakthrough.

In the privacy of the office of the counselor, a sympathetic woman, Sheila was finally able to tell the truth about what had happened. She broke down and wept. She said that it might have been her fault because she had refused her boyfriend, or because she had dressed too provocatively. Whatever the reason, she was desperately afraid it would happen again. It became clear that overeating was her way of becoming unattractive. If she remained fat, men wouldn't rape her, but they also wouldn't approach her and date her. Having this understanding didn't change things immediately for Sheila, but it eventually helped her to come to terms with what was driving her obesity. Ultimately, she took off most of the weight.

Sometimes I wonder why I did not become anorexic, as so many women have. Anorexics tend to be overachievers, perfectionists, and extremely insecure. For most of my life, I fit that description. I consider myself lucky not to be afflicted with that psychological disease where food becomes repugnant and your very life is threatened by a lack of nutrients. I've known girls who, although they are barely eighty pounds, look in the mirror and worry that they appear fat. They can literally starve themselves to death, driven by an unreasonable obsession that defies understanding.

The weight issue resides in mystery. It requires compassion on every imaginable level. It requires infinite patience, relentless attention, and prayerful treatment.

It's as though we view our bodies with our minds and not our eyes. And it's also as though we are prepared to dislike whatever we see. It becomes a basis for self-contempt, with consequences that follow us for decades.

If we can understand what's happening *when* it's happening, we have a chance to take positive steps. Without understanding, the challenge is overwhelming.

I know that my relationship with James left its emotional scars. I'm not at all blaming him. I'm simply saying that I jumped into the role as a caretaker when I was still immature. I played the part of the rescuer when I myself was lost at sea.

Psychologically and physically, I was intimate with someone I thought I knew—but I really didn't. I moved too quickly. I behaved irrationally. I didn't know what I wanted, yet I gave the impression that I did.

I thought I was helping James, but in reality I wasn't. I was enabling him. I was actually hurting him—and myself.

I was a confused teenager. But at that age, who isn't confused?

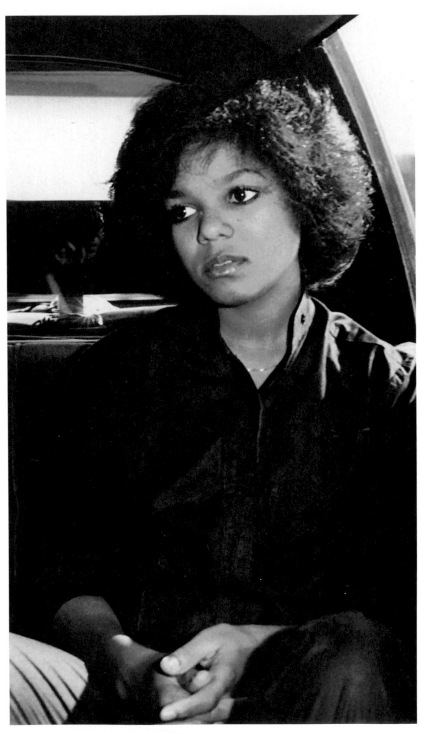

I am fourteen in a limo, feeling alone and overwhelmed.

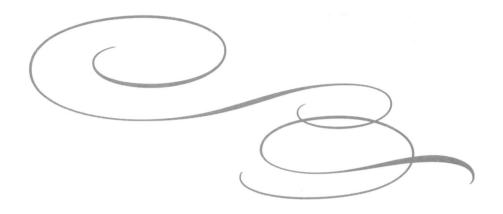

"Fantasy"

During my teen years, I spent a great deal of time in silence. The quick collapse of my impulsive marriage was nothing I wanted to talk about. I had neither an explanation nor apologies. I was young, and I was foolish, and I had made a bad decision. When I decided to get out of the marriage, I made a good decision, one based on a concept of self-care. I certainly didn't have a fully developed sense of self-worth, but I was slowly—very slowly—beginning to build such strength.

Even before I met James, I had begun dabbling in another area—artistic expression.

One day I wandered up to the recording studio that had been built in my family's backyard. I just started messing around. I'd watched my brothers work there for years. I myself had written poems and short stories since I was eight. I wrote my first song when I was nine and called it "Fantasy." But I never thought much about it. A few years later I began toying with the idea of writing music.

There was something about this rainy winter afternoon that had me fooling around at the keyboard. Joining words to music was new for me, but I liked it. I wasn't self-conscious, because I didn't take it that seriously. I was simply playing with thoughts and sounds in my head. I didn't think the thoughts were profound; I didn't think the music was great. I was merely expressing myself. The lyrics were all about my teenage-girl notions of loneliness and love.

I was able to work the mixing board well enough to lay down my music tracks and record my voice. And just as I didn't take the lyrics and melody very seriously, neither did I have much regard for my singing. I just did it. And after hearing what I did, I didn't even smile or feel especially fulfilled. The truth is that I didn't think about it at all. It was a few hours spent in solitude in which I was able to voice some feelings.

A few days passed, and I forgot about the music I had made.

Then one day I came home from school and saw that the door to the recording studio was open. The song that I'd written and recorded was being played at full volume. My first reaction was embarrassment.

When I got to the studio, I saw that Randy and my father were there.

"I guess I forgot to erase the song," I said.

"Why would you want to throw it away?" asked Randy.

"It isn't anything," I said.

"Who wrote the melody?"

"I did."

"And you did the drum and piano part?"

"I tried," I said.

"And the background vocals?"

"Are they out of tune?" I asked.

"No, they're in tune. And what about the lyrics?"

"They're kind of stupid, aren't they?"

"They sound pretty good. What do you think, Joseph?"

"Janet," said Joseph. "Did you really do this?"

"I guess so."

"It's not half bad," Joseph declared.

"I don't like it," I said.

"You can sing. I believe you can become a singer," he said.

"I don't want to sing," I said. "I want to act. I want to go to college and study business law."

My plan was to support myself as an actress. I greatly admired theatrical artists like Cicely Tyson. I had practically memorized Tyson's lines in *The Autobiography of Miss Jane Pittman.* I also loved classic actresses like Joan Crawford and contemporary ones like Meryl Streep.

"Acting is okay," said Joseph. "But you'll never make the kind of money acting that you will singing. You have talent as a singer."

"But singing isn't really something I want to do."

"Do you have any more tapes like this?" Joseph asked, ignoring my last comment.

"No."

"Doesn't matter. It's a good start. And it gives me a lot of good ideas about where you should be going. It shows me something I haven't seen before."

I didn't know what to say, so I said nothing. But deep down I didn't feel that it was wonderful. Joseph was taking an interest in a career for me—that part was okay. But the plain fact was that I was not being asked what *I* wanted to do. I wanted to complete junior high, then high school, then college. There was a world of learning I wanted to explore.

But before I could explain to Joseph why I wasn't interested in a singing career, my father closed down the discussion. It was his way. And that was that.

A few weeks later Joseph returned with the news: he had secured me a contract at A&M Records. I was set to do an album. I was all of fourteen years old.

I didn't want to do an album. I wasn't ready to do an album.

"Teenage artists are always the rage," said Joseph. "Frankie Lymon was. Michael was. And you're next."

But another part of me—a powerful part—didn't want to proceed with the project. Unfortunately, that part stayed silent. I was being a good little girl and doing what I was told. Don't get me wrong, I'm not whining. It's paid off well. I'm just telling you my reaction. And an essential part of the story is rooted in my inability to confront Joseph. Why, in fact, did I retreat so passively?

If I had felt better about myself, would I have spoken up and protested?

If I had not been afraid of Joseph, would I have resisted his plan?

If I had felt more secure in my body and in my soul, would I have found the strength to say "No, not now. I need to wait. I need to grow. I need to feel my way into the world and not be pushed"?

I'm still not sure.

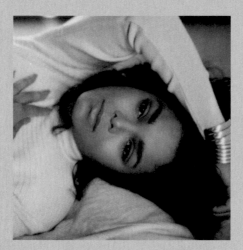

A private moment.

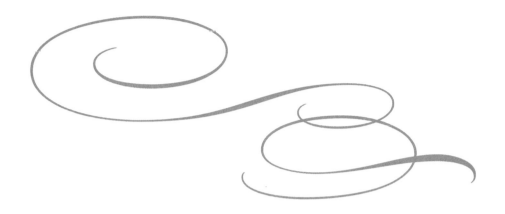

Start Anew

The truth is that in my career, I *was* pushed. I went along with the pushing. I went along with the program. I went into the studio and, as a young teen, began to sing under the guidance of producers Leon Sylvers III, Angela Winbush, and René Moore. Singles were released. "Young Love" was a hit with young people. I was about to fall in love, or what I thought was love, but my relationship was not as successful as the song.

I was still self-conscious about my image, my body. What would I look like on the album cover? How would I show my shape, which was still a source of uncertainty and, at times, of out-and-out shame?

I got the idea for a cover when I saw a photograph of Elizabeth Taylor taken early in her career. She was submerged in a swimming pool. You could see nothing but her face above the water; her body was hidden beneath the surface. I thought the pose was dramatic and I loved the fact that I could do the same thing and not have to reveal anything but my face. The record company hired the famous Hollywood photographer Harry Langdon, the sweetest man imaginable, to take the picture. He knew exactly what I wanted, but it was still a difficult shoot. With the photographer, his assistant, and other people around the pool, I was reluctant to take off my robe and stand there in my bathing suit. I was too shy to ask everyone to look the other way, so at a moment when everyone was distracted I quickly slipped into the pool.

We copied the original Elizabeth Taylor pose, and that was that. After Langdon was satisfied that he had gotten the right shot, I waited till everyone left before getting out of the pool. As a result, my first album cover as a solo artist would reveal nothing below my neck.

By today's standards, the record, titled *Janet Jackson*, did well, selling more than three hundred thousand copies. But by the standards of 1982, the year of its release, it did not. It was seen as a failure. And it certainly did not bring me any closer to the fame that had been achieved by my brothers.

The same is true of *Dream Street*, the follow-up album. At that point I was still a teenager going with the flow. In my family, smash hits meant everything. It wasn't enough to merely put out a good record. Joseph had taught us that anything less than number one meant failure. That lesson, though, hadn't really sunk in yet. I wasn't worried about reaching the top of the charts. I was just letting my father lead the way.

I knew that Joseph cared about success and that he cared about success for me. It took a while, but after *Dream Street*, at age eighteen, I also began to think about what it meant for me to care for myself. That was a different concept.

Slowly—very slowly—I was beginning to understand that if major success were to come, it would have to come on my terms, not my father's. If my early albums did just okay, as opposed to great, *I* would have to figure out why. If I wanted my music to reflect more of me, I'd have to put more of myself into it.

I wasn't afraid of falling short. I've always been pretty brave as a performer. I'll go out there and do what I have to do. But falling short while following someone else's agenda is frustrating and even infuriating. Falling short while following your own instincts is another matter. I could live with that. I could also see that, as I became more of an artist, my art needed to be self-reflective. I always had my own thoughts and ideas. But was I ready to put those things into songs or, better yet, into a concept album?

I thought so—but could I really step out and be myself? Could I be that brave, and that vulnerable?

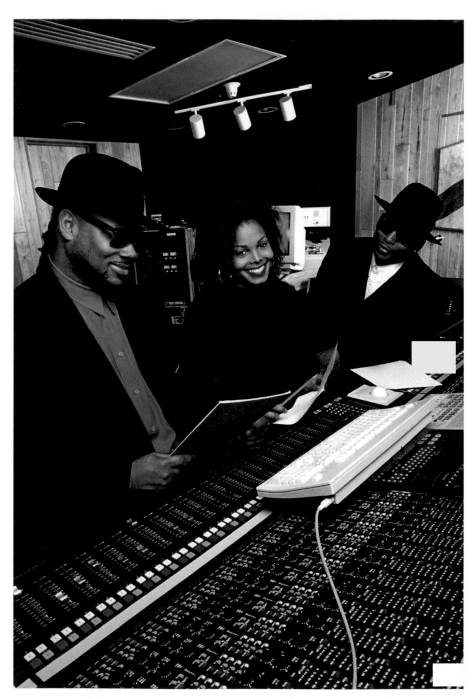

My other fathers, Jimmy Jam and Terry Lewis.

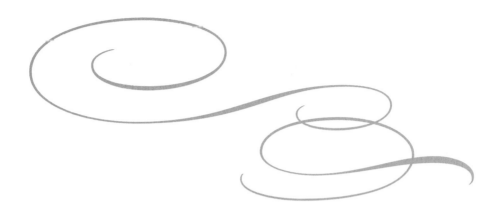

Control

At nineteen, I felt the need to take control of my life. I moved to Minneapolis to make the album *Control*, and everything changed. It was a watershed moment; my life was never the same again. The move had to be made, but it took everything I had to find the courage to do so. Yet it was exciting as well. I had admired producers Jimmy Jam and Terry Lewis for a long time. We had seen each other at different award shows and talked. I loved the music they were making and knew I wanted to work with them.

I was at an emotional dead end, however. Up until then, I'd depended on an authority that I recognized and respected. But I had also decided that the authority did not have the right answers. Remember, I had been an obedient child and was an obedient teen. So to figure out the next move on my own—and not on the basis of what others were saying—was scary.

I knew that I was leaving a big part of my childhood behind in moving to Minneapolis. I was losing the main connection to my father, which was about business, work, and career. Now I realized that to move forward, I had to start thinking for myself. I had to figure out where I was and where I wanted to go. I not only had to deal with feelings I had previously suppressed, but also had to put those feelings into lyrics and melodies. I wanted to write, not out of obligation, but out of passion. That meant identifying myself as my own person.

In short, I had to move on.

The first thing I felt was vulnerability. I felt unprotected. My father is a strong man, and whatever differences I may have had with his management style, I had been comforted by his strength.

"You're strong," said Jimmy Jam, who was producing the record with Terry Lewis. "You're stronger than you think you are."

The move to Minneapolis tested that strength. I was happy to be pushed by Jimmy and Terry. I was also able to push myself.

On one level, for all my show business experience, I had been brought up and sheltered in the suburbs of Los Angeles. In Minneapolis, I encountered a whole set of new challenges. Some were not pleasant. At one point, I was stalked by a group of guys on the street.

I had been heading somewhere when I noticed them following me. They began to taunt me and I began to feel nervous. But instead of running, I turned and faced them. I backed them down. I had wanted to run, but something inside me wouldn't let me do that. I had to confront them. It was a matter of self-respect and self-defense.

Those were the emotions I put into "Nasty" and "What Have You Done for Me Lately," key parts of the suite of songs that became *Control*.

Through Jimmy, Terry, and the other people working on the record, I made new friends in Minneapolis. One boy was a teenager, as I was, and he saw me as a sister. I liked him a lot. We'd have lunch together and sometimes walk through one of the malls.

I'll call him Todd. He was in his first year of college and was studying dance. He had recently gotten engaged to a girl back in his hometown. He described her as being "assertive."

"You mean sexually?" I asked.

"Yes," he answered.

"And that makes you uncomfortable?"

"I'd rather wait."

"Nothing wrong with that."

"She thinks there is. She says this is the move I have to make to prove that I love her and care."

"And when she tells you that, what do you say?"

"That I'm not ready."

"That sounds like a good answer. That sounds like you want to be serious about her before you have sex."

"She says that the only reason I'm hesitating is because maybe I'm gay."

"Is that true?"

"Maybe."

A long silence followed before either of us said anything. Then Todd began to speak about his older brother, who had come out to his parents two years before. His parents had flipped out and disowned him. They were religious fundamentalists and convinced that their son would burn in hell. I remember Todd saying, "I don't know which is the right move."

We kept walking and I waited a minute or so before saying, "Maybe it isn't a move at all. Maybe it's just you being you. You need to take your time and figure out how you feel."

"I feel a lot of different things," he said.

"We all do."

"And it's hard to decide. It's hard to say."

"You don't have to decide and you don't have to say. It's not like you have to make a declaration, especially since you aren't sure. It's complicated, and maybe it's okay just to live with the complications the way they are. I know that's uncomfortable."

"Janet, I'm really afraid of what my girlfriend will say if I keep putting her off. And I'm also real scared of what my parents will say if I tell them I have these mixed-up feelings."

"Sometimes parents are the right people to discuss our mixed-up feelings with, and sometimes they aren't."

"But I love my parents."

"That still doesn't mean that they're the right people to hear what's in your heart right now. They come from a different place and time."

"I don't want to disappoint them," said Todd. "And I don't want to disappoint my girlfriend."

"I understand."

"So what do you think I should do?"

We stopped walking and stood in front of a big department store. The mall was bustling. Everyone was in a hurry.

"I don't know, Todd," I said. "Maybe the best thing is just to wait awhile."

The actual song on *Control*—"Let's Wait Awhile"—was recorded before I met Todd. It's a song that I wrote with no particular person in mind. But after that discussion, I connected that song to Todd and millions of young people who might need encouragement to think rather than act, to pause rather than move. This album was the first time I got to really put so many emotions and feelings into words. It was very personal. And people could feel that when they listened to it.

Around the time of *Control*, when I was breaking off my professional relationship with Joseph, I received a letter from a girl who had liked *Janet Jackson* and *Dream Street*.

Dear Janet,

I think of us as friends, even though I know we're not. You're an imaginary friend, and that's good enough for me. We have a lot in common. We're about the same age and we both have older brothers who made big successes of themselves. One of my brothers is a heart surgeon; another is a professional athlete; and another runs a bank. There's a twelve-year gap between them and me. I'm the baby of the family. Our father is a military man and, as a child, we've lived all over the world—Japan, Germany, England, and about six different American cities. Living on an army base is strange, and living with a military dad is even stranger. It isn't that he doesn't love his children. He does. He loves us all very much. But he sees us as soldiers. He's our commander. He gives instructions that we must follow to the letter. If we don't, the penalties are really severe. He even treats Mom that way. Sometimes I wish she would disobey him—just so I could see what would happen—but she never does. She's afraid. So am I. And so are my brothers. They're all doing exactly what he told them do. We all have to be the best at what we do— and that's probably a good thing.

Except that I don't know what I'm really good at. My dad tells me I need to be a teacher and become the principal of a high school or the president of a college. I get good grades in school, but I'm not sure I even want to be a teacher. I'm good at drawing and am thinking of being an illustrator. Dad doesn't like that idea. If I date a boy my dad doesn't think has a future, my future with that boy is over before it begins. Or if I do find someone I like who passes Dad's test, next thing I know Dad is announcing that we're moving to a new base.

The strange part is that I actually like moving. It's been amazing to live in these different countries and cities. I've learned a lot about people and culture. I realize that I'm lucky to have these experiences and try not to take them for granted. I know that they've helped shape my life in a good way. But I also realize that every time we move, I leave a little piece of myself behind. There's a teacher I love that I'll never see again. There's a group of girls who were hard to get to know, and after getting to know them and forming a bond, I'm leaving. I'm always leaving and I'm always arriving and I'm always starting over again.

The friends I get to take with me are your records and a few books by the writers that I like. That's why I'm writing you. Whenever I move, I know I'll gain something, but I also know that I'll lose something as well. Do you use understand? I have a feeling you do.

I do understand. Moving beyond my father's reach was probably the most difficult thing I ever did. He had done so many good things for me. I also respected his discipline and sense of devotion to his children. Part of me didn't want to move to Minneapolis to make this record. But a stronger part of me—the part of me that realized I had to be my own person—managed to prevail. I thought I needed to take control.

I had been making small steps toward my independence for a little while. I remember when I bought my first car. I really wanted a jeep, like my brother Randy. My parents, especially Mother, insisted that I get a Mercedes. They saw it as heavier and safer. I went along. I was grateful to be able to drive such a luxurious car, but the car didn't fit who I was.

There were many wonderful rules in my family that I appreciate more today than I did at the time. We were given a sense of responsibility. One of the rules was that you had to be eighteen to have a car and you had to buy your own. Many of the kids I went to school with were given Porsches, Mercedes, and BMWs at the age of sixteen, as soon as they were able to drive. Then and now, I'm grateful that my family instilled in me the desire to work for and earn what was mine. I admit that it sometimes makes it hard for me to receive gifts. I'm more comfortable giving than receiving.

So much of my life is in my music and my videos. If you watch the long-form video of "Rhythm Nation," you'll see me getting out of a jeep and going to the club. That was actually my car at the time. By now I had sold the Mercedes and finally got the car that I truly wanted. I was in control.

I remember driving with my brother Mike in his first car, a Rolls-Royce. Mike reminded me of the family rule and said I would want my own car and independence when I turned eighteen, so I should make sure I saved my money.

My brother and I had a deep talk that day about a lot of serious subjects, and he gave me some advice. I wondered aloud when the world might end. Mike said we will never know when that day is coming and we should move ahead with our dreams and life goals. After that conversation with my brother, I knew that at some point I had to take control of my own life. That was a life-changing moment for me. I would have to be completely and totally responsible for me.

Control was the fulfillment of my very first dreams. I had finally achieved my independence. Years earlier I first heard the Time in concert. In the band were Jimmy Jam, Terry Lewis, Jellybean Johnson, Jesse Johnson, Morris Day, Jerome Benton, and Monte Moir. My mom was sitting next to me and saw how excited I was by the show. These guys weren't funky; they were *superfunky*, and brilliant musicians to boot. I fantasized about singing with a group like that.

When I got to Minneapolis, these were the guys I got to work with. I was completely comfortable because, in many ways, they reminded me of my brothers. They were good-natured and lived for music. Today when I watch the videos I made for *Control*, I remember being so energized by this new direction. I loved the new music and the new, independent life I was leading.

The success of *Control* was wonderful. The record was an international hit. My popularity soared, and I was suddenly seen as an artist in my own right, distinct from my family's success. I was gratified. But I was still under the illusion that total control was possible. This is the more complex part of the story.

Gaining artistic and management control was vital to me then and still is now. Working with Jimmy and Terry, I was passionate in writing songs, lyrics, telling my own story, and finding my own voice. I had to do that apart from my past. And yet, as I would soon see, none of us is really in control. If we continue to grasp for absolute control, we're going to end up in greater frustration and eventually in anger and even rage.

I'm still attracted to control, but I also know that an attraction can become an addiction. The more I have, the more I want. Just as there is no drink that will set the alcoholic free, no drug to liberate the junkie, there is no amount of control that will satisfy that kind of freak.

Only God is in total control.

Not me, not you, not anyone.

We make plans. We rehearse. We prepare. We seek good advice from good advisers. We organize our lives to maximize our potential. We seek to change in positive ways. We seek to grow.

And then here comes reality. Here comes an unexpected turn of events. A storm. A sickness. A betrayal. A promotion. We find a lost treasure. We lose a treasured friend, or a sister, or a brother. Our career soars, or our career sags.

We work to do the best we can and be the best we can. But can we control it all?

We can't. And when we finally stop trying, we realize the benefits of relaxation, acceptance, and peace of mind.

In many ways, whether in control or not, I was still preoccupied about body rather than soul. I knew that had to change.

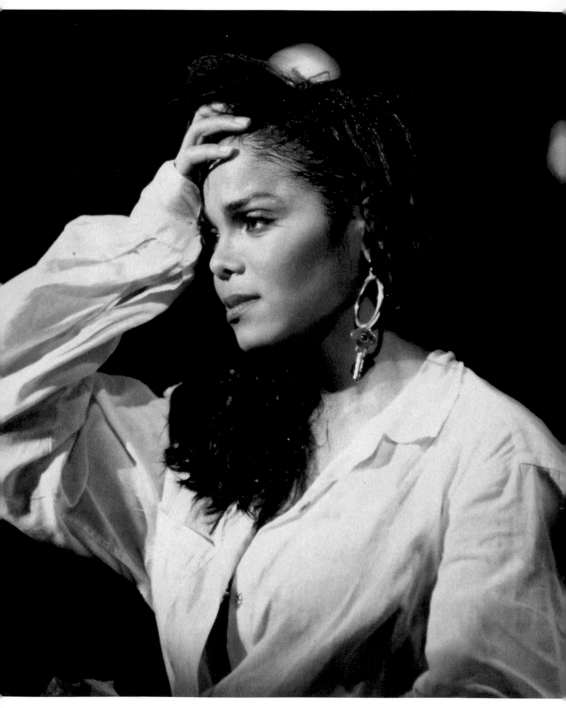

In concert for *Rhythm Nation,* feeling your love and feeling fraudulent at the same time.

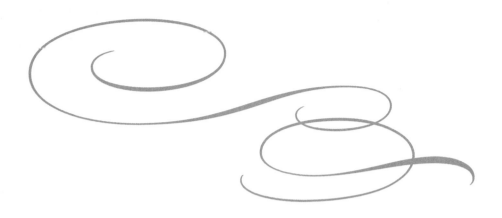

Rhythm Nation

As I approached age twenty-one, I realized that I had worried far too long about having a perfect body. I knew that the comparisons others had made between my body type and non–African American body types were unfair. I had internalized those comparisons and on some level had actually been traumatized by them. I wanted to be free of all that.

Before *Control* was released, a record company executive told me how he ordered the art director to take an X-Acto knife and slim down my image on the cover.

"You look too heavy," he said.

When it came time to do the "What Have You Done for Me Lately" video, the record people thought it was important that I appear thinner. That's all I needed to hear! I'd been told that my whole life, but at this critical juncture, with my career taking off, I didn't have the wherewithal to argue. Once again, I went along with the program.

I went to Canyon Ranch in Arizona with Paula Abdul, then a choreographer and friend. We shared a house and spent weeks exercising. I loved the natural beauty of my surroundings, but I hated the exercise. I've always hated it. Still, I was as motivated as ever to come out on top. I did the strenuous routine, the running, the hiking, the no-nonsense diet. I felt good when it was over. I enjoyed the compliments about my "new" shape. I shot the video and did in fact reshape my image. But at what cost?

It was a time in my life when I should have been enjoying success. But I wasn't. In many ways, whether in control or not, I was still preoccupied about body rather than soul. I knew that had to change.

I have friends who think that I grew up quickly. Others are convinced I grew up slowly. I believe both statements are true.

As a child, I worked in the world of adults. I had adult concerns and responsibilities. I could act like an adult. I could converse with adults. Indeed, I had an adult salary and certain adult responsibilities. But that didn't make me an adult. It wasn't until the end of the 1980s, when I began working on *Rhythm Nation*, that I began to view myself in completely grown-up terms. *Control* was a necessary first step in moving from childhood to adulthood. But it was with *Rhythm Nation* that I felt mature enough to address urgent social concerns. I also felt strong enough to ignore those business advisers who argued against making a record that dealt with issues like racism.

Looking back, I see that I made the decision as a confident adult, not a frightened child. I stuck to my beliefs, and not because I was stubborn or felt compelled to prove anything. I stuck to my beliefs because they were important to me. They were born out of my view of the world. I didn't see myself as an expert on social issues, any more than I see myself as an expert on more personal issues. At the same time, I couldn't ignore the blatant injustice in a country pledged to equality. I felt obligated to speak about troubling aspects of our society.

"We are in a race between education and catastrophe," I sang in "Race." I believed it then; and twenty-two years later, I still do.

I was very gratified when I saw my songs reach deep into the hearts of so many young people, living in every condition imaginable. I received a flood of responses to my music, much of it surprisingly personal.

Twins—a young man and woman—roughly my age told me about growing up in an impoverished neighborhood in one of our biggest cities. Their mom was a dark-skinned black woman and their dad a fair-skinned Dominican. She worked as a domestic and he was a part-time mechanic. The young man—I'll call him Dexter—had his dad's light coloring, and the girl—I'll call her Deidre—resembled her mother. So dramatic was the difference in coloring that not even their teachers believed they were twins. They carried their birth certificates wherever they went, just to prove it.

In school, Dexter received better treatment than Deidre. He attracted girls as well as the teachers' favors. Deidre was largely ignored. They both were interested in drama and were equally talented, but it was Dexter, not Deidre, who was accepted into the high school acting society. Deidre was every bit as attractive as Dexter, but her skin tone, even in this so-called enlightened era, held her back.

When they were teenagers, their parents died in a car accident and they were sent to stay with a relative who lived on food stamps in a tiny tenement apartment. She treated Dexter like a prince and Deidre like dirt. Brokenhearted, Deidre ran away to another city, where she was never able to escape the cycle of poverty. She worked in a factory and tried to complete high school at night. She lived in a boardinghouse run by a church group, but the church fell on hard times, the house closed down, and Deidre was forced to move in with a coworker. The coworker turned out to be a drug addict. Not long afterward, when Deidre's job was eliminated, she found herself living on the streets.

For years, Dexter searched for his sister in vain. He won a scholarship to college and it was in his junior year that, in his own words, he decided "to take control." He found an organization that dealt with missing children, and three months later they located

Deidre in a psychiatric hospital. Rather than deal with Deidre's problems, the inadequately funded facility kept her sedated on heavy drugs. Dexter valiantly fought the system and found a way to get his sister better care. He moved her to the city where he was attending college, and in time, she improved. She got her high school degree and was admitted to a business school.

When the twins wrote me, they were doing well and said, in an almost mystical way, that the musical background of their journey was *Control* and *Rhythm Nation*. The love of one sibling for the other had prevailed. Of course I was flattered and grateful that music could provide positive energy for anyone looking for motivation.

At the time of *Rhythm Nation*, my motivation was to open my mind and heart to subjects that were calling to me—problems I knew needed to be highlighted. I didn't want to appear glamorous or hip. I didn't want to draw attention away from the important matters at hand. I wore the *Rhythm Nation* uniform, an all-black outfit that symbolized the severity of the issues. It was the first time I wasn't singing about romance or relationships.

At the start of the project, I was still not comfortable exposing my body. In this sense, I continued to carry that self-consciousness about being too big that had followed me since childhood. I was happy to cover myself from head to foot in black.

Not long after the record came out, a woman my age wrote me that she had also decided to wear black every day for the next three weeks. For her, it was a protest against what she saw as sexual harassment.

I work in a field that's dominated by men, and in an office which is 90 percent male. Because I have a position higher than most of the men, there's a certain amount of jealousy. And because I am in my early twenties and not unattractive, I'm given an inordinate amount of attention. I've dressed conservatively, but I get whispered comments and stares almost every day. Of course those comments and stares make me uncomfortable, but there isn't much I can do. I've just continued with my job and ignored everyone who seems to be objectifying me. Well, last week my boss called me into his office and said that he thought my outfits were provocative. I had no idea what he meant—and told him so. "Your blouses," he said, "are too tight." Now I realized there were legal issues here, and I could have called an attorney to get advice. I might even have grounds for a complaint. But it took me a full year to find this job and another two years to rise to the position that I now hold. I need the money for both myself and my mother and I'm not about to get tied up in a legal hassle.

When I saw your Rhythm Nation, *Janet, the idea came to me: Wear a black outfit every day. So that's what I'm doing. Sometimes I wear a black pants suit, sometimes a black dress. When I come dressed in a black skirt, I make certain to wear a loose-fitting black blouse. When the men start questioning me about why I'm wearing black, I keep my answer short. "I like black," is all I say. I don't owe them an explanation. Actions speak louder than words, and I'm sure that my all-black statement is making the point. I'm going about my work with dignity, and I'm letting my boss know how I feel about his 'advice' to me. I don't foresee that I'll dress this way forever, but so far it's making me feel extremely good about myself. In fact, I never felt ready to fall in love until I had gained this kind of respect for myself. Now I've met a man for whom I feel great love, and I'm optimistic about our future. I had to join up in that* Rhythm Nation *to get things going!*

Rhythm Nation was a powerful time for me. I was developing a sense of self-esteem, partially because, through these songs, I was able to transcend some of my own problems and concentrate on societal issues. I was able to live with the criticism that I was moving away from the *Control* vibe that had brought me success. I was feeling a great deal of love.

One man who lived in a foreign country wrote me that the record spoke to him about the nature of assertiveness.

I'm twenty-four years old and never been able to tell another guy that I love him. The truth is that I have been in love with a man for a long time now. I was afraid to express my real feelings because—well, I guess I was afraid of being rejected. I act feeling vulnerable. What if he reacted poorly? What if, after pouring out my heart, he said he couldn't deal with me anymore? What if my confession of love led to the end of what has been a beautiful friendship? All these thoughts plagued me. I'm a lawyer and am trained to think defensively. Don't take chances. Cover your tracks. Play it close to the chest.

The man I love is also quite conservative. His job, like mine, is largely about making sure his clients are protected. Regardless, I felt that the time had come. I felt that the Rhythm Nation *was all about love, and I felt the* Rhythm Nation *spurring me on. I asked him on a date, made reservations at a romantic restaurant, and, after a glass or two of wine, finally said the words. "I love you." It felt great to say them. But also scary. He looked at me for a long time, and then began to cry. At first I was scared; I thought his tears meant that he was angry or repulsed by what I said. But when he took my hand and squeezed it, I knew that he loved me as well!*

Love is so strange. It feels so natural and good. Yet when it comes time to express it, I nearly choked on the words. I needed to assert myself. I needed to say what I felt. And now that I have, even more love has been released. It's wonderful.

To be a loving adult—to accept the responsibilities that come with a mature and generous love—isn't easy. I have no prescriptions for achieving that goal. Most of what I've learned is from listening to others and gleaning wisdom from the lessons of their lives.

A forty-year-old man I know is an only child who lives with his seventy-year-old mother. The husband/dad deserted them thirty years ago, and the mother has never gotten over it. She never dated another man, and she has always insisted that if her son left her, she would go mad. Nevertheless, he decided to go off to college. The day he left, his mother swallowed a bottle of pills and had to be rushed to the emergency room. My friend came back and attended a college close to home. He has not left since.

His love life has been stymied; he's gone through at least a half-dozen unsuccessful romantic relationships. He has spent years in psychotherapy, trying to understand this ironclad tie to his mother, and figuring out what it would take to leave her. For years he has been convinced that something is wrong with him—that some flaw in his character prevents him from going out on his own.

When he speaks of his mom, though, it is in positive terms. She reads a variety of magazines, newspapers, and books every day. She likes to discuss politics; she keeps up with the cinema; she attends lectures at the downtown library; and she has many friends whom she sees regularly. She hardly seems like an ogre. As you can imagine, though, my friend harbored a smoldering resentment for allowing himself to be captive. For many years—all through his twenties and thirties—he was simultaneously attentive to his mother and bitter in his behavior toward her.

A year ago, his mother, always in remarkably good health, developed a number of life-threatening physical problems and grew even more dependent on her son. He hired a nurse to help, but of course his mother wanted him to be by her side.

"Something shifted in me," he told me. "I realized that no

matter what people had been telling me—friends, psychologists, even well-meaning pastors—I actually felt privileged to be able to take care of Mom. Learning to love her, in spite of her demands, has been the challenge of a lifetime. To meet this challenge has been a triumph. Other people may choose to deal with the same sort of situation differently. Some might even accuse me of hiding out in her world for fear of entering a world of my own. I've looked at all these issues and decided that I'm not hiding. I'm seeing what sacrificial love is all about. I don't argue for the correctness of my decisions, and I don't expect anyone to agree with me. How people view me is none of my business. All that matters is that I've learned to love more deeply. This woman, for all her faults, has been the only way I could have learned these lessons. I thank God for her. The doctors say she has only a few months left. I cherish these months, and I know that when she is gone my life will be different. In many ways, it will be better—better because I stayed to watch how love can deepen."

The *Rhythm Nation* experience was a major learning experience for me. Ironically, though, it wasn't what I was teaching others; it was what others were teaching me.

"Dear Janet," wrote a woman I'll call Laurie.

I'm a young adult who grew up in a religion that believes in converting everyone to our strict doctrine. My mother has been a member of this church her entire life— as was her mother before her. The same was expected of me. I never considered anything else. I never questioned the church or rebelled against it. I attended a college founded by elders of the church, and I did extremely well. I married a wonderful man who, like me, was born into this religion. We decided to devote our lives to church and attend a theological seminary together. After graduation, we traveled to a foreign land where our mission was to show people our way—in our minds, the only true way—of approaching God. The year proved difficult. My husband became ill. Medical treatment was inadequate and we had to come home early. I didn't feel as though I had accomplished my goal; of all the people I had met, I hadn't been able to convert anyone. I questioned my powers of persuasion—maybe even my faith—and then fell into a period of doubt that led to depression.

I thought about those people I had met overseas. They were fascinating. Their culture was new to me and so were their various spiritual practices and beliefs. In my heart, I wanted to listen to them rather than make them listen to me. I wanted to understand their origins and characteristics. My husband felt the same. That's one of the reasons, I later learned, that he became sick. We were both there to teach, but when we got there, we realized our main mission was to learn.

Our church did not respond well to our report, which included some of the ideas I'm expressing here. They wanted converts. In their minds, our goals remained unfulfilled. We were chastised and made to feel like failures. As you could guess, that deepened my sadness and added to my confusion. Then, by chance, I was at the home of a friend who's a big music fan. I confess that I'm not. I grew up enjoying certain country singers, but that's about it. My friend had your song Rhythm Nation *playing on her stereo. I heard the words, "With music by our side, to break the color lines, let's work together to improve our way of life." The words went right to my heart. I felt the immediacy of what you were singing; the crucial need to break down all lines—color, social, even religious. For the first time, I saw what should have been obvious to me years before. It took a song, though, to make the obvious come to life. The love I was feeling as an adult woman was—and is—something I need to share. It's the love that counts, not the philosophy or theology or psychology behind the love. Love is simple. If it's pure love—if it's the compassionate all-encompassing love of God—it reaches outward. It touches others without making demands. It doesn't require membership and it doesn't charge dues. It's free.*

Maybe I'm naïve. Maybe I've misinterpreted your song. But that's the message it gave me. We're all part of the Rhythm Nation, *whether we live in the U.S. or Senegal, whether we're Jewish or Muslim, Baptist or Buddhist. So I've been marching on. My husband and I have found new work. We're still teachers, but we're teaching in a school that allows us to express the joy that comes with a love based on acceptance, not judgment, a love that isn't exclusive to one group or one set of beliefs. It's a love for everyone.*

Another story that came out of *Rhythm Nation* concerns twin girls, Kai and Keisha, who were leading wild lives. They disrespected their parents, neglected their schoolwork, and got into all sorts of trouble. Miraculously, the message of *Rhythm Nation* got into their souls. They took it to heart and turned things around. The transformation was amazing. They became serious about their studies and even graduated from nursing school.

They came to one of my concerts with the intention of giving me their graduation tassels. Their relatives told them not to, arguing that I'd never acknowledge them and would only throw the tassels away. The tassels arrived with a note from the twins. I was deeply moved. As a tribute to Kai and Keisha, I had them framed and met with them both.

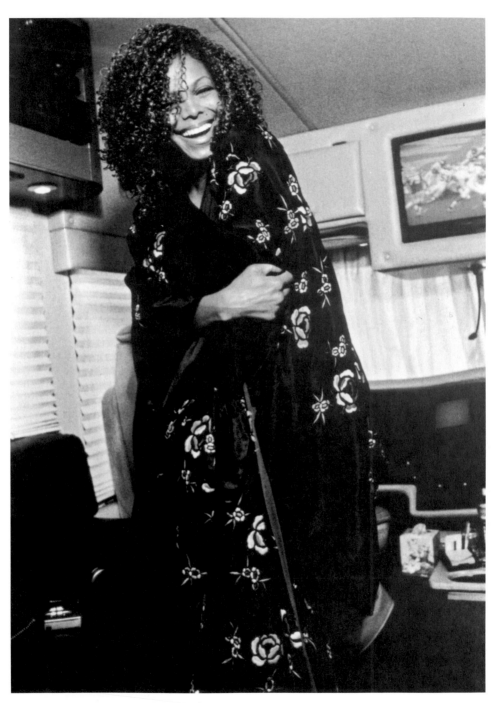

Hiding behind my smile.

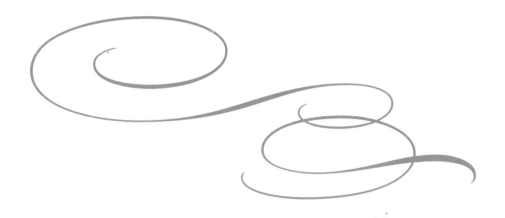

My Velvet Rope

In the last video for *Rhythm Nation*, "Love Will Never Do (Without You)," I had taken off the all-black uniform and danced in jeans and a halter top. The video was directed by Herb Ritts.

Herb was a lovely man who died far too early. He was a gifted photographer and filmmaker with a great eye for form and fashion.

Herb also spoke his mind. For most people that would be okay, but for me, given my extreme sensitivity, it wasn't always comfortable.

Years ago, when we were set to work together, Herb called me and, even before exchanging pleasantries, blurted out, "How's your weight?"

The question came suddenly, and I was taken aback. At the time I was feeling especially self-conscious about my body and didn't know how to respond. When I paused, Herb was even more blunt. "Janet," he said, "are you fat?"

"Well, no, not exactly."

"What does that mean?"

I didn't know what it meant and ultimately canceled the shoot.

Time passed and I wanted to work with Herb again. I realized it was my fault, not his, that I was so overly sensitive when it came to discussing my body. Besides, this time I knew that by no stretch of the imagination could I be called fat. I had gone on a stringent diet. I was feeling strong, and certain that many of the psychological challenges I had faced—involving lack of self-regard and worrisome insecurity—had been dramatically reduced. Herb planned for Antonio Sabato, Jr., and Djimon Hounsou to be in the video, men with remarkable bodies. But even that didn't intimidate me. I was starting to like the way I looked. Maybe even feeling free, at least during the shoot.

After the shoot, though, someone I loved said, "You can't be seen in public like that. You look nothing like your video, nothing like your television appearances. You can't go out." That contributed to my depression. I was too distressed to even go to a movie. I shut myself out from the entire world. There was the "Janet" that the public saw and the young woman who felt overweight. Despite the success and the public image, the private me felt I wasn't good enough. Unknowingly, I had surrendered to the programming of my childhood. Be aware. Be alert. Don't fall into your old patterns. It's hard to break the cycle.

I wasn't living life. Even though I am a homebody, it hurt me deeply to be told I shouldn't go to the movies because I didn't look right. I wish I had been able to cry. I realize now I was too numb. Crying would have given me some kind of release. Once again I kept it in inside.

I didn't answer, didn't argue. I simply absorbed the comment and, crazy as it seems, I didn't go out after shooting videos, especially if I had gained any weight at all. Between tours and records, I disappeared from the public.

When I appeared after *Rhythm Nation*, it was on the cover of *Rolling Stone* magazine, the same shot that became the image for the CD *janet.*

I thought up the pose when I was making the movie *Poetic Justice* with Tupac Shakur. I had just stepped out of the shower and put a towel around my waist when I walked to the mirror and placed my hands over my breasts. I thought it might look cool as a photograph if someone's hands were covering my breasts. It was just a fleeting creative idea. And I thought one day that if I ever had the courage to take a photograph like that, it might help me face the demons that were my body issues, my insecurities over how I looked.

Then came the day to shoot stills for *janet.* Patrick Demarchelier, the photographer, had me posing outdoors for hours. The session was about over, when I suddenly felt the urge to tell Patrick about my creative idea. All day I had been building up my courage to do so, convinced that the picture I had imagined was something I had to do. I believe in fighting the various things that scare me the most. Once Patrick and I moved indoors, I trusted him enough to take the picture.

I was so uncomfortable, though, that I had to ask everyone to leave the set. That was a battle, for sure. And though the photos were taken in private, it was being aimed at a large public. The conflict of my feelings, in being so shy but still understanding that creativity needs to happen, is at the core of who I am. It's ironic that some people feel I wanted to flaunt my body, when all I was really doing was trying to accept myself as a woman and express myself as an artist.

janet was extremely successful. The mood of the first song and its video, "That's the Way Love Goes," was relaxed and carefree. The groove was easy and fun, soft and seductive. It became the summer song of 1993. I had just turned twenty-seven and was ready to branch out. The record revealed who I was at that moment, presenting sensuality as an important and beautiful part of my being. I was optimistic. I was feeling free.

Yet within that feeling of freedom were seeds of discontent. I worked compulsively. There was a lot of pressure to achieve a certain look and, once I had achieved it, to maintain it at all times The photography, the videos, the world tour—the pressure was unrelenting to look a certain way during the entire process. In my determination to slim down, I overdid it—I underate and I abused laxatives to keep the weight off. In short, I didn't take care of myself. I want everyone to know: don't do it. It's not healthy. It's not worth it. It's not true you.

Writing, recording, promoting, and touring for *janet* was hard work, and I loved it. But I'm talking about four years of eighteen-hour workdays, six to seven days a week—nonstop work. Trying to look the way other people thought I needed to be, I was exhausted. No, I'm not going to point fingers and accuse anyone of manipulating me. I take responsibility for my choices.

During this same time, rumors began to spread that I had had a rib removed. The rumors were crazy, but they hurt nonetheless. The fact that I had achieved my look through discipline, not surgery, was important to me. It's no fun when people lie about you. And it can be infuriating when others pass judgment on you when they really don't know the truth, which happens frequently in the media today, especially with the growth of the Internet. That cutting remark, that carelessly cruel comment, can scar someone—especially a child—for life. That being said, when people are unkind, I remind myself to pray for them. I'm my mother's daughter. I'm a Christian. I can't be a hater.

Meanwhile, the relationship I was in that had brought comfort now showed signs of serious strain. Eventually it would collapse. I'm legally prohibited from detailing this relationship, but, in truth, I entered it of my own free will. Again, it was a choice for which I take responsibility. I don't believe in making excuses. Nor do I believe in blaming others. In the end, that does no good.

I began to understand that my view of people—especially some who were very close to me—had not been as clear as I had imagined. Doubts crept into my mind. Self-condemnation crept into my heart. I was assaulted by harsh thoughts: *How could my judgment have been so poor? How could I have been so naïve? How could I have fooled myself into believing that I was actually a good entertainer?*

I was unrelentingly critical of everything I did. This not only caused weight fluctuations; it also caused my moods to change a lot.

There were times around *Rhythm Nation* and *janet* that I fell into deep despair. I internalized what I was told about the difference between my public image and how I really looked. It reminded me of my childhood admiration of my sister Rebbie. It's strange how the public was complimenting my appearance while at the same time I hated what I saw in the mirror. I would literally bang my head against the wall because I felt so ugly. I was inconsolable. To the outside world, everything seemed perfect; now everyone knows that it wasn't.

No matter, I forged ahead. The work ethic that had been such an essential part of my upbringing served me well. After the *janet* tour, I disappeared from public view. What should have been the happiest experience of my life left me lost. But why? My music was well received. My popularity had risen dramatically. Yet the lesson I was learning had not come into focus—I hadn't found my essential core. The concept of the true you was still many years ahead of me.

I now understand that my inability to voice my pain had to do with the way I was raised. *Keep your problems to yourself.* I was afraid of burdening others with my anxieties. I didn't want to be a whiner. In a later song, "In Better Days," I wrote, "I don't want to waste nobody's time."

My escape was to do what I've always done—work. The demands of show business both helped and hurt me: helped by keeping me active; hurt by allowing me to sweep the dirt under the rug. I acted as though nothing was wrong.

I forged ahead. I had a new album to prepare, new songs to write, dance routines to learn, a world tour to plan. I expressed my emotional confusion in terms of a metaphor. I called the project *The Velvet Rope*. The meaning is open to a wide range of interpretations. To me, the rope represents a kind posh prison in which I found myself. Psychologically, I couldn't break free from a place of darkness to a place of light—so I wrote about it.

Literally, the velvet rope is the barrier that keeps partygoers outside a nightclub from getting to where they want to be. You can look at these partygoers in many ways, however. It's those people who simply want to have fun but are unable to gain admission to the fun room. It can also be those people who are seeking relief from the weight of their problems, and people looking to belong. To get beyond the rope—at least the rope that exists in my imagination—requires, in the words of the songs, not putting people down, but rather freeing ourselves from feelings of hatred and oppression.

One writer called *The Velvet Rope* "a dark masterpiece." Of course, I appreciated the highly complimentary term *masterpiece,* but at first I was taken aback by *dark.* I didn't—and still don't—see myself as an artist who operates in darkness. My aim has always been to put a smile on your face. But I realized that that very pressure—to entertain at any cost, to be positive, to act carefree, to present a public face in contrast to my true feelings at the time—was contributing to my psychological confusion. I had to work through my fears through music. That was my way of taking care of myself.

"I'm trying to get past my own velvet rope," a fan wrote.

I'm the youngest of three sisters. They've always seemed to be in the VIP section of life—and I've always felt on the outside. My sisters went to Ivy League colleges. I went to a state university. They both joined exclusive sororities. I never did. They attracted wealthy and handsome boyfriends. I struggled in that area. After college, they married and began families. At twenty-seven, I really haven't gotten over my shyness and feelings of inadequacy. I dress in ways that hide what most people would consider a good figure. I don't spend money on expensive haircuts or cosmetics. In fact, I don't spend money on myself at all. At work, when I'm asked to attend the managers' meetings, I take a seat in the back. Something keeps me from sitting with the "cool people" up front.

I could go on and on, but I know you get the point. I usually don't write letters like this, but when this velvet rope incident happened, I knew I had no choice: Friends asked me to meet them at a club over the weekend. I love music, I love to dance, and I was excited to accept the invitation. When I arrived, I saw it was one of those ultra-hip places with a bouncer holding a clipboard standing in front of an actual velvet rope. My friends were already in there. I told that to the bouncer, but he didn't care. My name wasn't on a list. I was about to turn away and just leave. I hate those situations when I have to prove something or assert myself. I hate confrontations. But just as I started leaving, the door to the club opened wide. They were playing your "Together Again" from The Velvet Rope. *The music poured out into the street and straight into my heart. The rhythms danced round and round my head. I felt something I couldn't even name. But instead of leaving, I headed straight to the door of the club. I actually leaped over the velvet rope! I'm a good athlete, so I made it with room to spare, but jumping over velvet ropes is hardly my style. By the time the bouncer knew what to do, I was in the club, dancing to "Together Again" with my friends who greeted me with open arms.*

During my *Velvet Rope* days I had no choice but to face what were some serious blues. In spite of the fact that people responded positively to the record, I continued to withdraw inside myself. I didn't really want to call my condition "depression," because I've never been comfortable with labels. I knew, though, that no matter what the term, I was being assaulted by a negativity that threatened to overwhelm me. I sought the advice of friends and professionals. I've said it before but need to say it again—I'm not a preacher or a psychologist. All I can do is summarize the good counsel given to me. These are ideas that came from people who were genuinely concerned about me and offered loving help.

Depression is serious. It has a life force, but also the potential to be a death force. It has an energy that is powerful and capable of imprisoning you. You can't ignore it and hope it'll go away. You can't simply say "Oh, I'll get over it." It isn't a matter of willpower. You have to recognize its immense strength. You have to fight it, as you would any other enemy.

There's a big difference between being depressed and merely feeling temporarily depressed. Please don't let your depression define you. It can be one of many elements that impact your life on any given day. It's good to acknowledge it when it's there and then decide how you will fight it. Depression is so real and dangerous that it must be figured out. Whatever your path, please don't ignore it. Use every resource, your faith, or a mentor, and don't be ashamed to get professional help if you're not making progress. There is free help available online, there are twenty-four-hour crisis call centers, but no one can help you if you don't open up. I've heard people say, "Oh, eventually it will pass." Sadly, that isn't always true. I'm still grieving about teenagers who were clearly depressed and committed suicide recently because they felt trapped, with nowhere to turn. I wish I could have talked to every one of those kids. I know how real depression is, and that's one reason why I've written this book. Speaking openly about depression takes away its power.

Depression wants you to feel hopeless. But there are other resources that live within our hearts—prayer, resilience, joy, gratitude, love, compassion for yourself and your emotional fragility—that will surface and give you not only hope but strength. Still, sometimes depression is so overwhelming that we can't find our resilience and strength on our own. At such times we need others to show us that those qualities still live inside us.

Just when you're convinced that this is the day the cloud is starting to lift, it returns for another day, another week, another month. That's reality. Just as we have to be patient with others, we have to be patient with ourselves and the brutal mood disorders that assault our sanity. We have to be patient with our impatience. The cloud will lift. It always does, but not always when we need it to.

By now you know that I've always worked hard, and I'm grateful for that. In the past, I've used my work ethic as a defense against depression. I'm the kind of person who pulls herself together and goes out and does what needs to be done. I know it isn't easy and that, yes, even getting out of bed can seem impossible. But work for me was sometimes a blessing and a way to avoid dealing with my problems. I now accept that work alone will not conquer depression, not entirely. For many years I continued to struggle with overeating. I realized that even though my life was different in many ways, I had so much more in common with other people. I began hearing about others who grew up as the only person of color in their community, feeling isolated in their community: people who felt like outsiders; people whose families were successful, but their success didn't transfer into their own lives; people who felt less-than. I would wonder. I would ask about discrimination they had experienced; in some cases yes, in others no. But it did not surprise me to see how many people connected with what I was expressing in my music.

I was recently in Paris and met a young man of color who warmed my heart when he told me that *The Velvet Rope* had saved his life. I don't know his entire story, but I felt the truth in his eyes. He was shaking as he approached me and when we talked, even though it was briefly, with very few words, our hearts connected. He told me that he was using the Internet in a wonderful way. He said he was building a website where people could come and just have a dialogue about their lives, about their pain. What he gave me was precious. I felt such joy to know that the music I had written in 1996, as I opened up, has helped others deal with their own lives and struggles with depression. It's so good to talk about our troubles together.

Work helped. It always does. But it didn't chase all the blues away. I continued to struggle, and struggling often meant overeating. The comfort of food seemed to ease the discomfort of my moods. I received more meaningful comfort, though, from family, friends, and fans who, having sensed my discomfort in *The Velvet Rope*, opened up their hearts.

So many things can block the true you. For example, racism is very real and powerful. My thoughts go to Reg, who had a privileged background and didn't feel authentically black.

"I wasn't even sure what 'authentically black' meant," he said, "but that didn't matter. I knew I lacked authenticity. Other guys were from the projects or the streets. Even if they came from middle-class neighborhoods, those neighborhoods were predominantly black. Once again, I felt like an outsider. When I was rejected for membership in a black fraternity, I retreated into a shell and stayed there for the next four years. I made good grades and graduated with honors, but I never got past the velvet rope."

Reg's next move was to Europe. He lived in Paris, learned French, and got a job as the assistant to the publicist of a famous designer.

"No matter how well I spoke the language and did my job," he said, "I still felt inauthentic. I loved the culture, I loved the work, loved the people I met, and yet I couldn't shake this notion that I was trying to be something I wasn't."

Reg stayed in France for five years. From there he went to China, where the economy was booming and the opportunities were unlimited. His amazing facility for language allowed him to learn Chinese in only six months. His past experience paid off. He began his own firm, specializing in publicizing Chinese fashion designers in Europe. He did extremely well and soon had beautiful apartments in Shanghai, Paris, and London. Magazine articles were written about his success. His services were in demand, and Reg became a celebrity in his own right.

"I flew from one country to another," he said. "I was never in a city for more than three days. There were exciting meetings with exciting personalities, exciting plans for the future. Now when I went to a fashion show, I was escorted to a prime seat in the first row. There was no velvet rope I couldn't get past. I was wearing velvet sport coats and flying in private jets. But you know what? Inside I still felt empty. I heard that song you put on *Velvet Rope* called

'Empty' and realized it was about me. It was about someone who had a fantasized romantic relationship on the Internet. There were all sorts of men who were attracted to me and I to them, but that nagging self-doubt deep inside kept me away from real romance. Despite my resources, despite my high profile, when it came to intimate relationships I lived in the world of make-believe. I was afraid of going out there and getting rejected. There were sexual encounters, but most of them short-lived and even anonymous."

Things went downhill for Reg. He developed a cocaine addiction that nearly did him in. He fell apart and nearly lost his business. When he completed a long period of rehab, he spoke to me of the experience.

"My entire life has been about filling up that famous hole in the soul. It turns out not to be a hole, though, but a bottomless pit. Prestige, drugs, luxury apartments—you name it. None of it gave me what I lacked. Self-respect. Self-love. I had to be stripped down to nothing to realize that the running had to stop. I had to look at myself for who I am, accept who I am, and find, through the grace of a divine power, an appreciation for myself, flaws and all."

I wanted to know what rehab was like for Reg.

"There was group therapy," he said, "as well as individual therapy. I did a lot of journaling and also attended twelve-step meetings. But the biggest eye-opener for me was this simple realization: I hadn't been taking care of myself. And, to be honest, I didn't even know what it meant to take care of myself. That had never been part of my life. When they spoke of surrendering and admitting that I was powerless over the mess I had made of my life, I didn't know what they were talking about. How could I surrender? I was the one who had graduated college, moved to France, moved to China, learned both languages, built up a thriving business. I had the power. I was in control. And I could never give up that control. 'When you decided to enter rehab,' said one of the counselors, 'you decided that this job—repairing your soul and gaining mental health—was beyond your control. You knew you needed help. You surrendered the care of yourself to others. You admitted that you needed others to teach you self-care.' That surrender and admission were monumental. Because the paradox is that most of us need others—other people, programs, and prayers—to show us how to care for ourselves." Yes, and how to love.

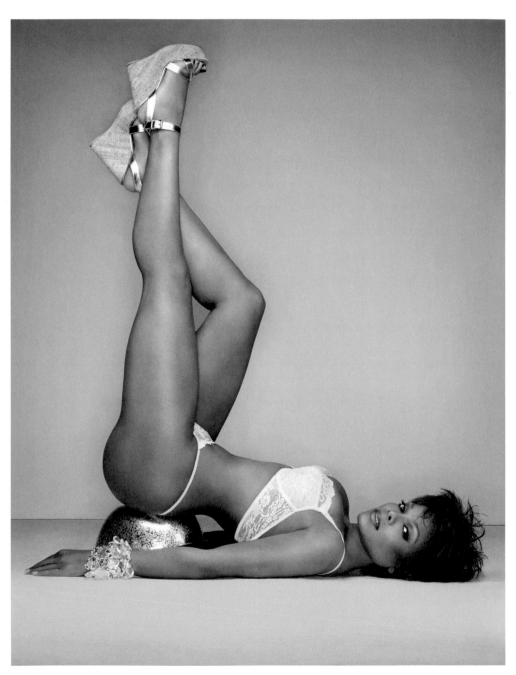

A picture no one has seen until now.

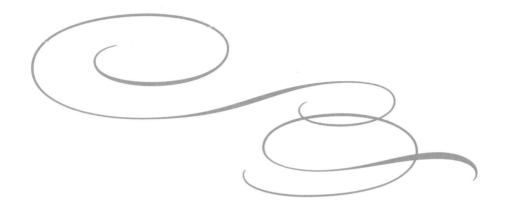

Soul Support

Jermaine Dupri was my boyfriend for many years and remains a close friend. He made me feel beautiful in a way that no one else ever had. He praised parts of my body that I didn't consider attractive, assuring me that they were beautiful.

"All of you is beautiful, Janet. Don't be ashamed of anything," he told me.

If I told Jermaine that my booty was too big or my thighs too fat, he never failed to say that I was wrong.

"I love you the way you are," was his constant mantra.

During those days in 2006 when I ballooned up to 180 pounds, Jermaine was always positive, supportive, and loving.

To be reassured by a friend is a gift from God. Often others see the beauty in you while you, conditioned by hypercriticism, see only flaws.

Long ago, a friend gave me a helpful exercise. He said, "Look in the mirror until you see something you like."

"There's no part of me that I like," I said.

"No matter, stand there until you find a part that you do like."

I cried in front of the mirror for a long time, still unable to find a part that looked right to me. I wanted to bolt.

"Keep standing there," my friend insisted.

Finally, glimpsing myself from the side, I liked the look of the small of my back. I liked the way it curved.

"Good," he said. "You've started the journey. There'll be other places you'll learn to like."

To honor that one place, I had a tattoo inked into the small of my back, a permanent reminder that positive self-regard is possible.

One day I answered the phone and heard someone I cared about crying on the other end. She said, "I'm moving out on him. He's critical of every part of me. Whatever positive picture I had of myself is gone. I'm moving far away from him and starting a new life. I'm moving to a new coast, a new city. I'm starting over."

"Okay," I said, and kept listening.

"He's like a drug that messes up my mental health. I tell myself that he can't do me any good—and I know that's true—but I also know he needs me. And I need him to need me. All that neediness is insanity. We keep running around in a circle like dogs chasing their tails. He cheats, he lies, he gets caught, he apologizes, he begs for forgiveness, he convinces me, he gets me back, and then he makes me crazier than ever. I gotta get away. I gotta put three thousand miles between him and me."

I was silent for a moment and then I said, "If that's what you need to do, go ahead and do it. But you also need to look inside and not simply run away from dealing with the issue."

A month later Greta called from the East Coast. She had moved, found an apartment, and gotten a new job.

"Jan," she said, "I'm flying out for the weekend."

I didn't want to ask her why, but I knew. The pattern continued. In fact, it still *does* continue.

I believe we're either moving forward or moving backward.

"That applies almost to everything," my friend explained. "We can change cities, countries, and hair colors, but nothing changes until we figure out how to change our attitude and belief system. We move backward when we keep doing the same things and expect a different result. We get discouraged and fall into despair. Superficial external moves—like a new wardrobe or a new apartment—just have us moving from side to side. Different scenery, same sensibility. Be careful, because all of that may be just smoke and mirrors, because it's not going to cure your pain. But to move up, to gain a higher consciousness and a more effective way to deal with our problems—that requires faith. Faith in something bigger than yourself."

I found faith in God as a child when my mother brought us to the Kingdom Hall of the Jehovah's Witnesses. My mother leads a rich spiritual life. I have beautiful memories of her sitting by the beach, reading her Bible, while La Toya and I roller-skated on the promenade overlooking the ocean. As I grew older, I no longer followed every aspect of Mother's beautiful faith, but I have never wavered in my belief in a loving and compassionate Christ. My mother exemplified that love and compassion. It really didn't matter to me that her scriptural journey was different from mine. The beauty of her spirit said everything. In my own journey, I've tried to find my personal understanding of divinity. I've listened to preachers, teachers, rabbis, ministers, monks, priests, and anyone else who seems to be connecting to the source of love. When it comes to the spiritual life, I'm committed to having a closer one-on-one relationship with God every day.

A man I know recently went through a nightmare divorce and spoke to me about the spirit of generosity.

"When I discovered that my wife, the mother of my three young girls, had met another man in another city, my heart shattered into a million pieces. My mom had left me and Dad when I was ten, so you can imagine my reaction when my wife said, 'You no longer interest me. You no longer excite me. I need to move on.'

"At first I didn't believe her. Our marriage had seemed good, our children are terrific, our lifestyle is comfortable. Where were the indications that something was wrong?

" 'The indications were subtle,' she said, 'and you're too insensitive to notice them.'

" 'Was it sex?'

" 'The sex between us was decent,' she said, 'but not spectacular. I want spectacular.'

" 'Well, can't we work on it? Can't we go to a sex counselor who might help us discover how to make it spectacular?'

" 'I don't have the patience,' she let me know. 'Besides, it's far more than sex. You box me in. You cramp my style. You fill up the room with your presence and there's no room for me.'

" 'I'll work on that,' I replied. 'I see that as a problem, and I promise I'll do my best not to dominate.'

" 'You've tried before, and you failed.'

" 'I'll keep trying.'

" 'It's too late.'

"And so our discussions went nowhere. When I questioned her about her new man—what he looked like, what he did for a living—I got no response. It was none of my business. When I questioned her about how in the world she could destroy a young family like ours over an impetuous romantic fling, she said, 'You call it a fling. I call it love. In this beautiful relationship, I'm finally allowed to be who I always wanted to be. I'm no longer suffocated or intimidated. I'm flowering as a woman with her own mind, purpose, and talent.'

"The more she spoke, the more devastated I became. There

was no ambivalence in her attitude. She wanted out—plain and simple. Because I'm close to the girls, and because I knew our girls desperately wanted us to stay together, I considered using them in my determination to win back my wife. But thank God the therapist I was seeing said, 'That's the worst thing you can do. It's called triangulating. Instead of pleading your case to your wife, you use your children to plead for me. That puts them in a terrible position. All that does is confuse and frighten them. They're confused because they're taking on an adult role, and they're frightened because they aren't certain that, in that role, they can make a difference. If they don't—and chances are they won't—their feelings of failure are tremendous burdens for them to carry. Whatever you do, don't put your children in the middle of these emotional negotiations.'

"I listened to the professional. I kept my children out of the fray as best I could, and instead I pleaded my own case. I lost any semblance of self-respect and basically just begged my wife to take me back. I wrote her letters, emails, text messages—you name it. I cried crocodile tears and literally got on my knees. I didn't know what else to do. I love this woman and couldn't imagine life without her. But as you might expect, the more I begged, the more repugnant I appeared to her.

" 'You're weak,' she said, 'and the last thing I want is a weak man. Just move on with your life. Put this behind you.'

"How could I do that, though, when she haunted my days and my dreams, week after week, month after month? Someone said the pain will pass. 'You're mourning the death of a relationship.

And the mourning period, although long, can't go on forever.' It sure felt like forever, though.

"Next came a period of bitterness and vitriol on my part. I wanted to hurt her—if not physically, certainly emotionally. I wanted her new man to cheat on her and leave her as she was leaving me. I wanted her to lose her job, lose her looks, lose her peace of mind. I hated myself for these cruel fantasies, but I couldn't turn off my negative mind. How to stop this destructive pattern of thought? After all, I married the woman; I once loved her deeply and probably always will.

" 'Pray for her,' said my minister.

" 'Pray for her!' I exclaimed. 'After what she's done to me and our girls?'

" 'Yes,' he repeated. 'Pray for her. Pray for her happiness, her well-being, her spiritual and material prosperity.'

" 'If I do that,' I said, 'I'll be faking it.'

" 'Faking it is fine,' he said, 'because in the course of faking it you will eventually come to a place where you mean it.'

" 'I don't think so,' I said.

" 'I do,' he replied. 'If stimulated by positive thoughts—especially thoughts that involve the betterment of others—the mind moves on. The mind heals itself. But to do so, the mind needs to move from stale energy to fresh generosity. Generosity of spirit.'

"There was that term again—*generosity of spirit*. It became my mantra. I railed against it. I didn't want to be generous; I wanted to be vengeful. Revenge felt good. Revenge meant closure—and it also meant victory. If I could hurt her as she hurt me, I'd feel less hurt. Praying for her felt false. Wishing her harm felt real. And yet I knew that, as the mother of my children, the more comfort she felt in her heart, the more comfort they too would feel. I had to grow beyond my own pain and consider how to avoid inflicting further pain on my kids. I had to move my mind in a positive direction at a time in my life when dark negativity was surrounding me. Move beyond darkness to light. Move beyond pain to healing.

"I heard a man on television talking about wounded hurters and wounded healers. 'When you get cut,' he said, 'you either want to pass on the pain or help people who have suffered themselves. You think that by passing on the pain you lose the pain, but, in truth, that only prolongs the pain. There's only one way to break the cycle, and that's to head into healing mode.'

"I believed all this healing business. I was determined to implement it. And live according to the laws of love and forgiveness. But just as I adopted that high-minded attitude, she hired a divorce lawyer, a pit bull disguised as a man. Without going into the gory details, he made demands—in her name—that went beyond the bounds of reason. If I had acquiesced, I'd face financial ruin. So much for the spirit of generosity. I returned to my original state of rancor. If she was getting a pit bull to attack me, I'd hire a Rottweiler. Attack, assault, intimidate, destroy. All-out war. With the kids in the middle.

"My wise friends kept saying, 'Stop and think. Take a deep breath. Pray for wisdom.' I took their advice, and rather than hire a Rottweiler, I spent a couple of weeks listening to the music and reading the poetry that helped quiet my mind. When I came out of this period of meditation, I decided to invite my wife to lunch.

She accepted. The day of our get-together, I called the most loving and generous of my friends for words of encouragement. I spent a long time that morning looking at pictures of our daughters. In the car driving to the restaurant, I went over all the things in my life for which I'm grateful—my health, my children, my connection to a spiritual source of strength. When I arrived, she was already there. 'Gee,' she said, 'I've never seen you look so relaxed.' That set the tone. We had a reasonably good discussion and—thank God!— I actually convinced her that my financial ruin was not in the best interest of anyone, especially our children. We agreed that working through overzealous lawyers would do no one any good. I assured her that I would be generous in the settlement. I wanted her to be comfortable and I wanted her to be happy. She was astounded by my attitude. After she had hurt me so deeply, she was convinced that I was going to hurt her. 'That's why,' she said, 'I hired such an aggressive attorney. I was afraid of what you might do to me finan- cially. I was afraid that you'd want to punish me.' Her motivation was fear—the one emotion that, unleashed, can destroy anything and anyone.

"In the final analysis, our divorce has been the most difficult chapter in my life. I have to live with the undisputed fact that the woman I love has rejected me for another man. I'm still haunted by thoughts of what I could have done to change things. But 'could haves' and 'should haves' only perpetuate more misery. And I'm not interested in misery. I'm interested in movement—positive spiri- tual movement from self-pity to self-assertion. I am who I am. My now ex-wife is who she is. I can't get her back. I can't make her love me. All I can do is fill myself with more love—and hope that she does the same. All I can do is minimize the destructive elements and maximize the creative ones. Out of this emotional debacle, can I be a better and more attentive dad, a more compassionate and understanding human being?"

My friend's story inspires me. I say that because most of us have lived through the collapse of romances and relationships. I know I have. It's hard not to dwell on everything that went wrong. I'm one of those people who tend to blame themselves when things don't work out. I need friends to remind me to keep moving forward. There's nothing to gain by going over everything that went wrong. That's stale energy. Fresh energy gets me going; stale energy leaves me stuck.

A beautiful lady—I'll call her Inez—told me the sad story of how her husband had left her for another woman. When I asked why, Inez said, "I had gained weight. He said that he no longer found me attractive. He said that if I really loved him, I'd lose the weight and make myself sexy for him. He reminded me that when we got married, I had a perfect figure. 'That's the figure I fell for,' he said. 'I'm not into fat girls.' 'I'm not a fat girl,' I replied. 'I'm a full-figured woman.' With that, he laughed in my face and walked out the door. This was a week before my thirty-fourth birthday, which I wound up celebrating alone. In the following weeks, I overate like crazy. I medicated myself on chocolate. When I learned through friends that my husband was with another woman—a *slender* woman— I started eating even more. I piled on the pounds and was on the verge of becoming dangerously obese.

"When he filed for divorce, I broke down. Crying, eating, unable to sleep, I went to see a counselor, a wonderful woman, who told me, 'You need to get healthy, not for your former husband—but for yourself. Your husband has failed the loyalty test. You're a big-boned woman and you're never going to be reed thin. But reed thin is not healthy, and reed thin is not you. Go to a nutritionist and find a healthy program that works for your body and your lifestyle. Get moving.'

"I got moving. I found a nutritionist who had helped other women with my body type. He designed an eating program that was neither instant nor miraculous. It was slow but steady. Over six months, I dropped significant weight. My confidence was back, along with my self-esteem and my figure. By then my ex had broken up with his skinny girlfriend. When I ran into him in the mall, he was amazed at my appearance. He was all over me with compliments and even come-on lines. 'I know you did it for me,' he said, 'and, baby, it's working me like crazy.' I just smiled and walked away. When he called that same night, I didn't even bother to pick up. I had moved on."

Movement for me also means exercise. I'm like most everyone else when it comes to getting in shape: I don't want to do it. I need motivation. Sometimes motivation comes in the form of looking in the mirror. Sometimes it comes in the form of a firm commitment to meet my trainer. But even if you like what you see in the mirror or don't have a trainer, that doesn't mean movement toward exercise isn't possible. I've been given wonderful advice from wise professionals; their insights about what it takes to get moving have made a big difference. They have taught me to . . .

Set reasonable goals. Don't bite off more than you can chew. A little bit goes a long way. If that means spending only ten or fifteen minutes a day, then spend that time and don't berate yourself for not spending more. Build up slowly. Ease into a rhythm and let that rhythm carry you.

Be open-minded about the form that suits you best. Don't do the exercise you feel you *should* do—do the exercise that you actually might enjoy. Some like to run, or walk, or spin, or dance, or stretch, or play soccer or softball or basketball or volleyball at the beach. Doesn't matter. Movement is movement. Make what moves you—music, competition, solitude—part of your exercise life.

I was taught that consistency is the key. Find what works and keep at it.

Have fun.

My trainer, Tony Martinez, always turns my workouts into games. He'll put together an obstacle course for me; he'll get me to throw a basketball back and forth to him, quicker and quicker, until my heartbeat is accelerated. We have timed runs. He gets me laughing like a little kid. He keeps it fun. He's always encouraging. Tony is a major part of my fitness program and my ability to stay connected with my own true me. He inspires me and everyone I work with, too. He'll bring fitness equipment to rehearsals so I can keep my stamina up when we're preparing for a show. He keeps us moving even when it's as simple as adding a game to our workout sessions. He makes me laugh. I know that not everyone can afford to work with someone of Tony's great talent. Thus one of my dreams is that Tony will be able to share his gift with the world in the future. If I didn't have Tony with me, I don't know where my body would be right now.

It's one thing to lose weight with a nutritionist, as I was so fortunate to do with David Allen's wonderful help; it is yet another entire effort to keep that weight off, to be fit, to stretch, to be strong, to have definition, to keep a strong core, to always stretch. And as you get older, it certainly doesn't get easier. Tony has given me the tools and support to be healthy and fit.

I get discouraged. I get lazy. I think to myself, *Enough! This exercise routine has gotten old and I've gotten bored! I just want to eat what I want to eat and forget about everything else because it tastes so good.* It's like a drug addict or alcoholic who drinks or uses one time and thinks he or she can handle it. And even with all the support I have, the work continues. I think to myself, *I earned the right to have this reward meal. I wanna eat what I wanna eat.* But the difference is, we all know we have to eat. It's true that we must eat to live, not live to eat. But we must do it in a healthy way.

Since you're reading this book, you likely know all about the internal voice that whispers to you, urging you to slip back. That voice is strong and never goes away entirely. I hear it just as I hear the voice that tells me that I'm not the person—the artist or friend or daughter—that I should be. To quiet those voices of negativity, self-doubt, and self-loathing, I must first acknowledge my inability to turn them off completely.

They've been there too long and they're too deep a part of who I am. All I can do is ask them politely to turn down the volume. I can live with those voices if I recognize that there are other positive voices that tell me that, as a child of God, I'm loved, I'm valued, and I'm capable of achieving balance in my life. I can learn to eat well. I can exercise. I can express gratitude for the simple act of being able to breathe in and breathe out. I can move away from darkness and depression to light and hope. I can be happy with who I am, not what I should be, or what I might have been, or what someone tells me I must be.

I am me, the true me; you are you, the true you—and that's good. That's beautiful. That's enough.

. . . as a child of God,
I'm loved, I'm valued, and
I'm capable of achieving
balance in my life.

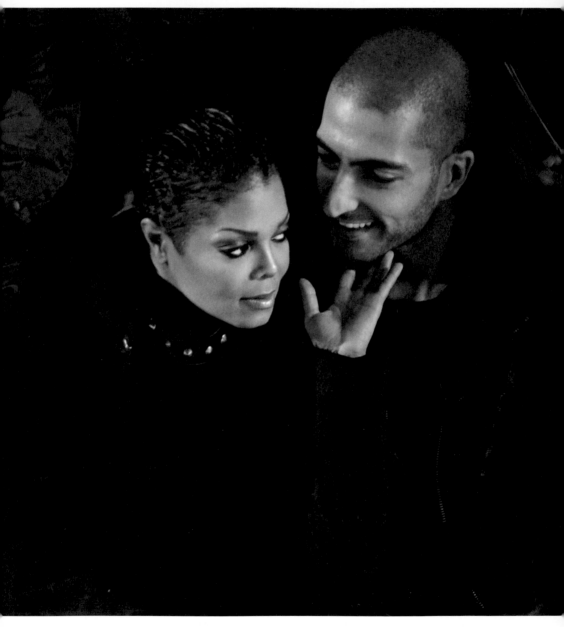

My life today in Paris.

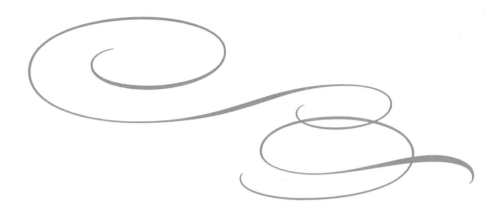

Loving My Life Today

I've never been happier. I'm finding peace; I'm growing my faith; I'm feeling confident and strong. And I'm in a wonderful new relationship.

It's funny, though, how rumors continue. While I was making two films with Tyler Perry—*Why Did I Get Married Too?* and *For*

Colored Girls—some said I had given up music. Meanwhile, in this same period, my "Make Me" was a number-one dance hit and my performance of "Nothing," the theme song from *Why Did I Get Married Too?*, was the top video on iTunes.

The truth is that I'll never give up music. I love it too much. I have great energy and passion for all the arts. And I want to do it all. There will be more records, more films, more dancing, more television, more books.

I'm often asked if there will be children. That's up to God. I love the idea of being a mother. I love being Auntie Janet to my nieces and nephews. They've given me a great sense of giving and caring. Children are my heart.

My heart is young. I believe you can know and enjoy what is happening at this very moment as well as innovate and bring something fresh to the party.

I realize that my life has been shielded from many things. I was protected by my family, especially my mother. We were encased in a very special bubble. Yet we were fully aware of the world—for good and bad—in which we lived. For example, there has never been a time free of the ugly specter of racism. Like all blacks, we have seen bigotry firsthand. I want to avoid specific anecdotes; many have suffered far greater indignities and pain than me. Comparisons don't help. Let's just say that as recently as 2010, doors that had opened for others were closed in my face, just because of the color of my skin.

I feel enormous gratitude for those brave artists who came

before me and paved the way. I'm speaking of Lena Horne, Eartha Kitt, Sammy Davis, Jr., Dorothy Dandridge—the list goes on and on. They are my heroes. The indignities these geniuses suffered were far more obvious than the racism we encounter today. Today's racism is more disguised and subtle. But it's there—and it hurts on many levels.

My growth depends on faith, as it must for everyone else as well. My spirit of generosity and selflessness also depend on faith. I'm grateful for the comfort that my work provides. I'm grateful for the privileged life that I lead. But I realize that it's the spiritual life that sustains, that nourishes us. In the early morning hours, when I read my Bible, when I pray, when I talk to Jesus, I'm no longer haunted by remorse. I know that the mistakes I've made are in the past; they're gone, forgiven, and no longer cause for guilt or shame. I'm looking forward, not behind.

Yet as my life goes forward, part of my past remains eternally present. In dedicating this book to my brother Mike, I want to pay tribute to his beautiful spirit. Not a day goes by that I don't think of him, his smile, his laugh, those little private jokes between us. He taught me so much. We were as close as close can be. It's still difficult to speak of him, still difficult to realize that he's gone. I can only look at his photos when we were kids. I turn off the TV or radio when anything about him is discussed. As I said on the BET Awards show, "To you, Michael is an icon. To us, Michael is family."

Our family is focused on Mike the brother, the son, the father, the uncle, the loving soul. I focused on him on July 2, 2010, when, for the first time in two years, I gave a full concert. It was at the Essence Music Festival in New Orleans, a city that has been the scene of so much bravery in the face of tragic loss. I dedicated my closing song, "Together Again," to Mike. Friends said that there wasn't a dry eye among the more than thirty thousand folks in the audience. I know my eyes were wet with tears when I sang these words, thinking of the joy my brother brought into my life and the lives of millions . . .

Everywhere I go
Every smile I see
I know you are there
Smiling back at me
Dancing in the moonlight
I know you are free
Because I can see your star
Shining down on me.

I know that the mistakes
I've made are in the past;
they're gone, forgiven,
and no longer cause for
guilt or shame. I'm looking
forward, not behind.

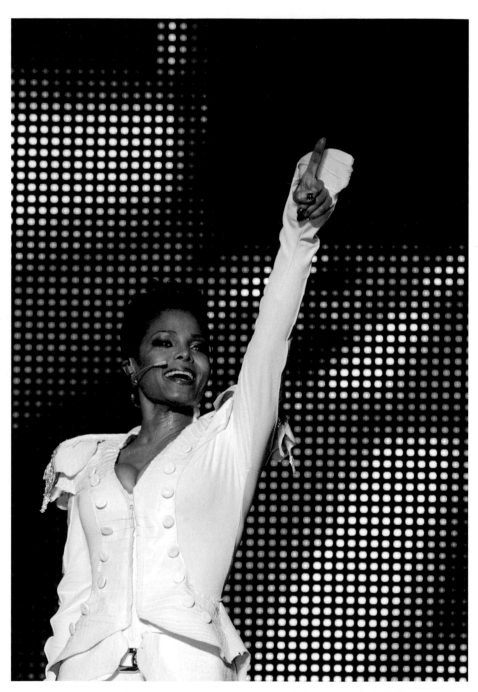

Back on stage. Finding and living, my own True You.

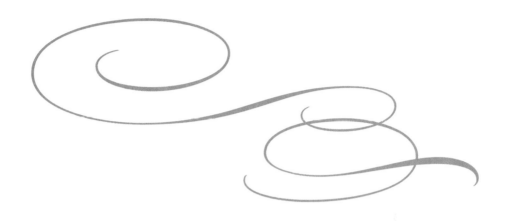

Meet David Allen,
My Nutritionist

Eight years ago I weighed more than a hundred and forty-five pounds and was concerned about an upcoming video shoot. My makeup artist, Timmy B., suggested I see the nutritionist David Allen. "The man is a genius in his field," said Timmy, "and I know he can help you."

Because I'm essentially shy, I'm always a little reluctant to reveal personal information to a stranger. I decided to go meet with David, but I had some reservations.

The interview was extremely thorough. David asked whether I was on any medicines. I wasn't. He questioned me about my health history, whether I had problems with blood sugar or high blood pressure. I had neither. He wanted to know whether my energy was good and my sleep patterns were consistent. I was given basic tests for possible blood, gastrointestinal, and adrenal issues.

I had been on many diets, but nothing worked long-term. In that way, I was very much like other people who struggle with weight. I'd be determined for a while, find a plan, follow the plan, see some results, get bored with the plan, and stop. I told all this to David, and was surprised by his response.

He told me to stop working out. He told me to stop everything I thought would work. Not only did I drop all of the weight I needed to lose, but I gained a perspective on how to live my life and be healthy.

What David gave me wasn't a diet, it was a way of life.

I was relieved that David didn't grill me about my past eating habits. I didn't want to list an inventory of every wrong thing that I had consumed.

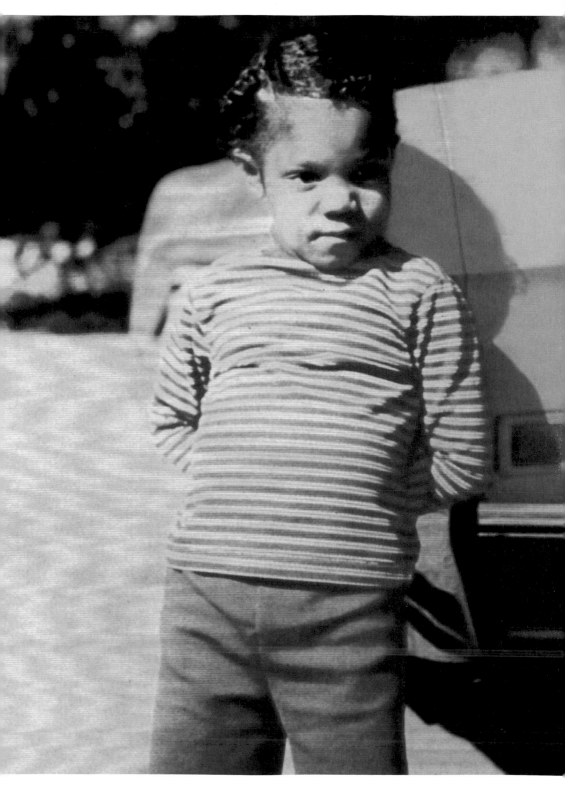

Baby me.

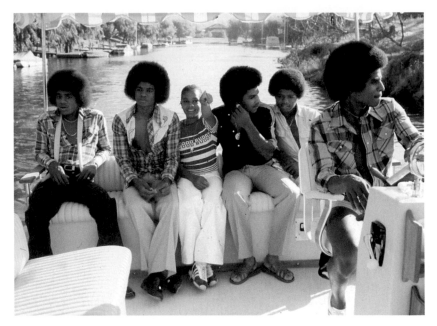

A beautiful day with my brothers. Whenever they were on tour, I missed them so much.

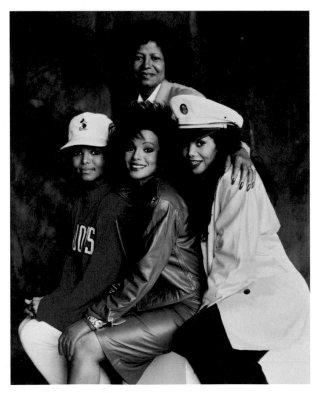

With my beautiful sisters and beautiful mother.

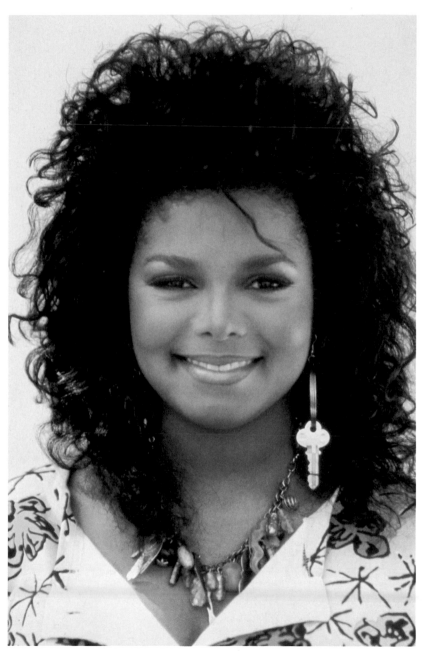

Battling with my weight issues. During "When I Think of You."

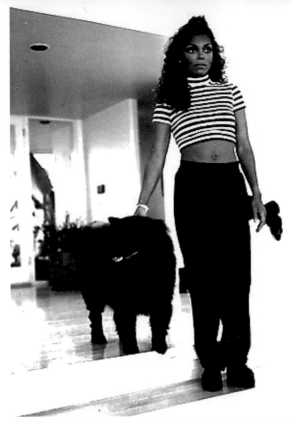

Here with Buckwheat. On my way to the MTV Movie Awards, the same day I got home from the hospital. If you look closely, you'll see I'm still wearing my patient ID bracelet. Things aren't always the way they seem.

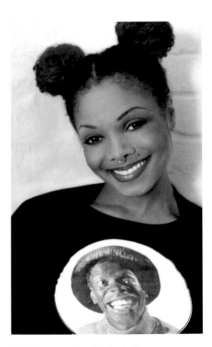

I still have this shirt of Jimmy. Beautiful memories.

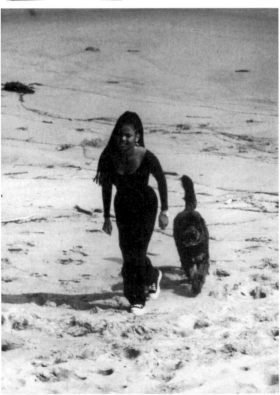

At the Malibu house with Puffy. The beach is a gift that reassures me that everything will be all right, no matter how I'm feeling.

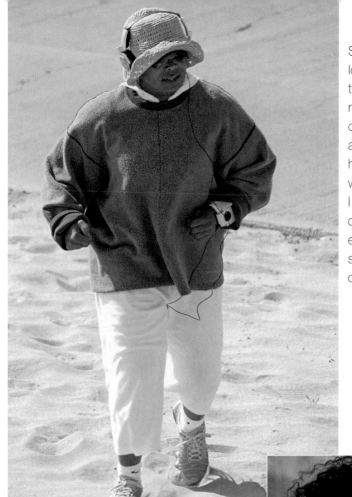

Some people in the media loved sharing these pictures of me with you. What no one asked, and no one knew, was that I actually had more endurance here than in other images where my weight is down. I was running 5 miles a day in the sand and I was eating very clean. The stress wouldn't let me drop the weight yet.

Fighting so hard to keep it all together when you're on the verge of falling apart.

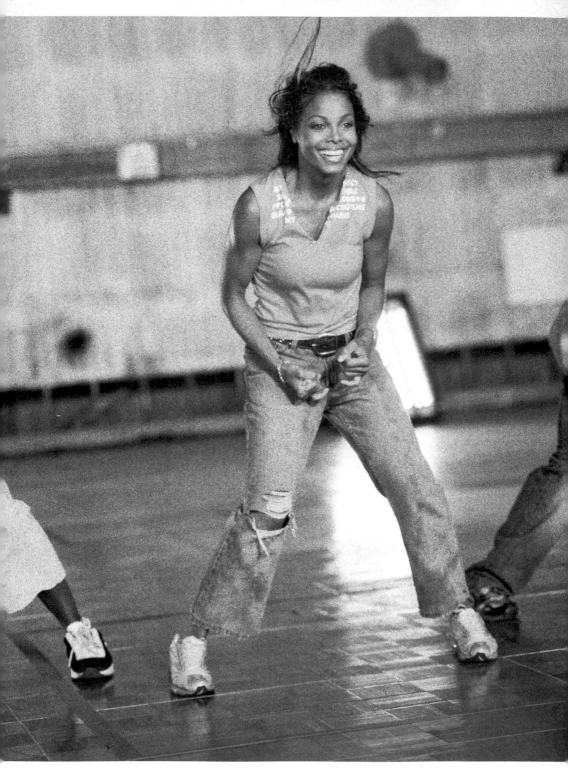

In shape and ready to tour. All the exercise in the world doesn't matter
until you find the True You.

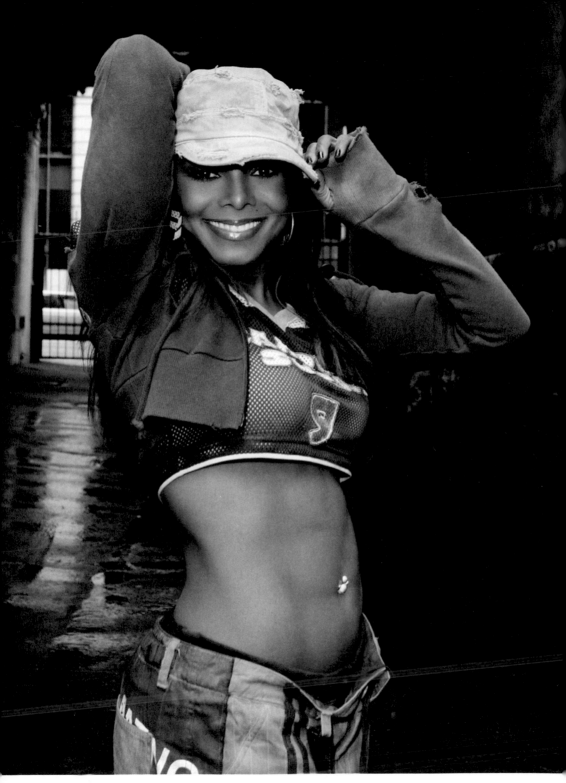

I was shooting a video for *Damita Jo* when this picture was taken.

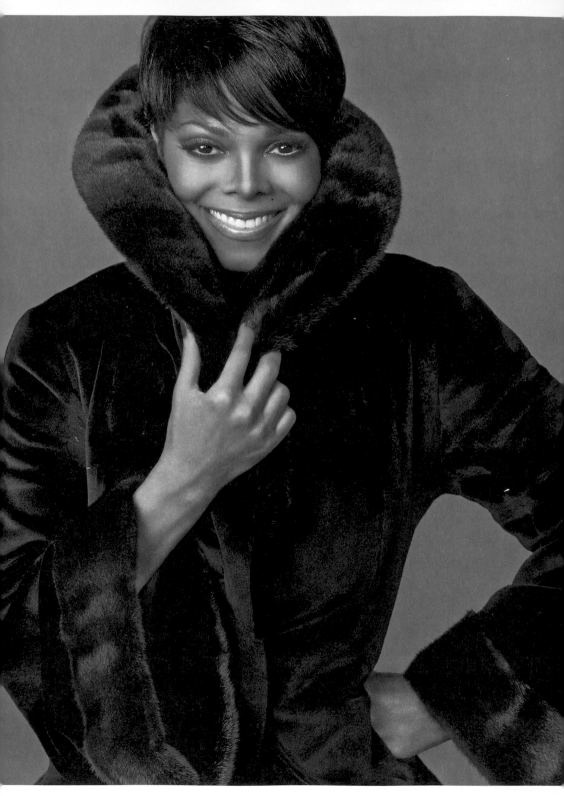

My first Times Square billboard. Blackglama.

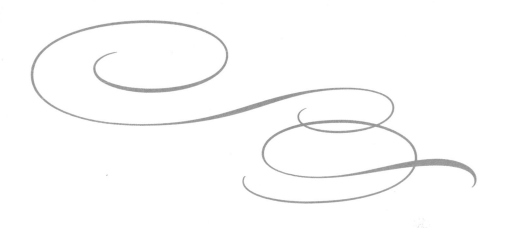

Afterword
It's Not a Diet!

By David Allen

When I saw that Janet Jackson had scheduled an appointment with me in October 2002, I was excited. I'm a fan. I expected her to show up with an entourage. I was delighted—and impressed—when she arrived alone. She was sweet, soft-spoken, and refreshingly down-to-earth. I liked her immediately. She was dressed in simple sweats and wore a baseball cap. She seemed a little camouflaged to me. Her answers to my questions were very short, usually a word or two. I also noticed her texting. I didn't feel as though I had her undivided attention. With all my clients, first impressions can tell me a lot about their personalities and habits. It is important to understand how they perceive and process the stresses of their life. This can be very helpful in moving forward and making subjective observations on an individual basis.

Janet seemed asymptomatic. Her main interest was in losing weight. In between the mandatory questions, I began to get a feel for her lifestyle. I identified her as an undereater/overeater, as many high-achievement professionals are. That description might sound weird, but it is a very common phenomenon. Many people will undereat during their day due to their intense work ethic and their focus on children and family. They will skip meals or allow too much time between them. Then they will transition to the evening hours, at which point they will overeat, indulge, and continuously snack. In the case of Janet, she often neglected to eat during the day. She usually missed breakfast. She worked relentlessly, starving herself until the cravings took over. Then she would binge on whatever meal she could fit into her overloaded schedule.

For example, we had an on-location appointment during one of Janet's video shoots. After sitting for about three hours waiting to see her, I met her in her trailer and asked, "Have you eaten anything?"

"No, I haven't eaten all day," she said.

I told her that she had to eat something, but before she was even able to have a cup of tea, they called her back onto the set, where she worked for another three to four hours. Many people can relate to being similarly stuck in lunchtime meetings or getting so bogged down with their day that they "forget" to eat or don't have the time to grab something sensible.

Janet had a long history of dieting. Her body weight and fat composition had yo-yoed throughout her life. Janet had struggled with her body image since a young age.

I don't believe in diets. I don't offer a diet. I look at diets as prescriptions for failure. A diet has a beginning, middle, and end. At the end of the diet, the dieter inevitably reverts to the lifestyle that caused the weight gain. To maintain a healthy weight requires maintaining a healthy lifestyle. That's the heart of my approach.

I concluded my initial consultation with Janet by asking her to complete as "homework" my extensive packet of lifestyle questionnaires that focus on food preferences, personal habits, gastrointestinal function, adrenal health, sleep habits, hormonal balance, cognitive function, and all major physiological systems. I also requested that a comprehensive set of specific blood tests be done for Janet. I planned to see her in one week, at which time she would start her new journey.

"Let me go over all your material, Janet," I said. "Let's meet in a week and I'll recommend a plan."

I try not to be judgmental with anyone. I also try not to dwell on the past. I'm a today-is-the-first-day-of-the-rest-of-your-life kind of guy. If you spend a lot of time going over everything you've done wrong, you wind up feeling guilty and defeated before you get started. If you want to feel good, look good, and gain health and positive energy, then give up your regrets, forget the past, and look toward a positive present and a healthy future.

It is during the second meeting, after I have reviewed all of a client's questionnaires and testing results, that I am able to design a plan that will strategically address his or her individual needs. In Janet's case, we started her on our 21-Day UltraCleanse program.

"I'm not sure I can make such a radical change," she said.

"Sure you can," I said encouragingly.

And she did.

Two weeks later, she had lost eight pounds, and seemed upbeat.

I asked her, "Are you feeling deprived?"

"Not really," she answered.

"The minute you feel deprived, you're in danger of reverting to old habits. How is your energy?"

"Greater than normal," Janet said.

"Wonderful," I said. "Are you still feeling those extreme lows?"

"No, not at all."

"Then we're on the right track."

By November, Janet had lost twelve more pounds. I was glad, but also a little concerned. She was traveling a great deal and had been missing meals. There was another challenge: the holidays. Thanksgiving was around the corner.

I told Janet to enjoy the holiday and eat whatever she liked. She was a bit surprised by my advice. But just remember this: Thanksgiving is one day, not an entire month. If you have your dinner out, don't take anything home. If you have your dinner in, make sure your guests take all the leftovers. Enjoy the day as a special occasion when we express gratitude for our blessings. That occasion is so tied into food that there's no way around it. Come Friday morning, though, gently slip back into the new lifestyle that you have come to accept and enjoy.

When Janet came to see me after the holidays, she had put the weight back on. In the first three months of the new year, she was in what I call the fifty-fifty zone. Half of her was committed to the new lifestyle; half of her wasn't. Because I had seen what Janet had done when completely focused, I knew she could do it again. But I also knew that she was slipping back into old ways. This was her yo-yo pattern. The winter was rough, and by the time summer came around she was up to 150 pounds, her new set point. By "set point" I mean the weight to which her body metabolism tended to gravitate. It is that comfortable point at which your body fluctuates up and down two to four pounds, no matter what you do. This is something a great many people have experienced.

I could tell Janet was discouraged. But I knew she could do it. The name of the game is trust. I wanted Janet to trust me so I could instill new habits into her life. No matter what her situation, the fact that she was meeting and speaking with me proved her sincere desire. Her effort was always there. Her heart was always in the right place. She was looking for light, looking for a way to stay strong. This can be a very crucial point in making a life change. Life is about struggles and its ups and downs. I try to keep my clients focused on moving forward. Weight loss can be very difficult because people are usually making a drastic change and for that level of commitment they expect dramatic results.

In order to achieve long-term results and happiness you must change your expectations. I use the following example: If you went to work for a week and put in twenty hours of overtime and when it came to payday your boss gave you only fifty dollars extra and asked you to work extra next week, your answer would be "I quit!" I relate this story to weight loss—you work extra hard while making numerous changes and sacrifices, and then get on the scale to discover that you do not get the reward you expect.

What do you do? *You quit your diet.*

This is why you must make the decision not to be on a diet but to change your life so that you can achieve the desired outcome.

Later in the second year that we worked together, Janet became serious again. Filming was on the horizon and she wanted to shed weight. She embraced the new lifestyle with new determination. We got her back to eating balanced meals that along with snacks were designed for her work/stress load. She was to concentrate on getting sufficient sleep. I think I drove her crazy with my insistence that proper sleep is key. Without the right amount of rest, we lose our emotional and physical equilibrium; we're vulnerable to all sorts of volatile energy and moods, and to physiological imbalance.

The bottom line is that the second time around, Janet focused on proper nutrition, and she went from 153 to 128. And she looked terrific.

During this period, I explained to Janet the importance of increasing caloric intake. (This surprised her. "You mean I should eat *more?*") But when the body is under intense stress and an increased workload, you need more calories for balance, along with additional nutrients. It is during this period of increased activity that many people tend to cut back, which is a real mistake.

Janet and I had contact at least five or six days a week during this time. She'd text me questions; sometimes she'd express doubts or insecurities about maintaining her weight. I'd always text her back, letting her know that my confidence in her was unshakable.

Then one day I got a call.

"I'm sorry, David, but I have to take a break."

I knew that meant no more daily contact. I respected her decision, wished her well, and let her know that she was free to call whenever she wanted. I wasn't going anywhere.

When lifestyle change is not fully adopted, it is very common for people to stop their "diet" and return to old and familiar habits. That is why it is so important to understand from the very beginning that you are not on a "diet"—you are embarking on a lifestyle change and adoption of healthy habits that will bring you balance. I can say one thing with the utmost confidence: here at David

Allen Nutrition we have learned from experience that though clients drift away, they later return because they realize that during their time with us they felt and looked their best.

Janet:

During this period, I was going through personal challenges. The part of me that wanted to medicate myself with food took over. I remember David saying that food is the most powerful drug of all, the one drug you can't give up. You can't stop eating. If you're a compulsive eater, the addiction can kick in at any meal. A hot biscuit. A piece of cake. An ice cream bar. Anything can you set off. I was set off. I was off all plans; I was lost in a world where I ate whenever and whatever I wanted.

It was sometime after Christmas of 2005 when Janet called after a long absence. I was elated to hear from her.

"David," she said, "don't be angry at me."

"I wouldn't ever be angry at you, Janet. That's not my style."

"I've gained weight," she said.

"We all gain weight from time to time."

"A great deal of weight," Janet said.

"Why don't we talk about it in my office instead of on the phone?"

"I'll call for an appointment after New Year's."

Janet:

When I walked into David's office, I could see the shock on his face. I had ballooned to 183 pounds. I had no choice but to level with him.

"David," I said, "in four months I have to be ready for photo shoots and public appearances. Can we do it?"

David didn't hesitate. "Of course we can do it."

This was serious. Janet had reached a dangerous level, one she had never experienced. That in turn had caused an array of health problems, including weight gain.

I was upset for her. More than ever, I wanted to help her beat this demon that kept assaulting her peace of mind. I wanted her to put the problem behind her. I was determined to have her permanently adopt a balanced lifestyle so she wouldn't have to go through this torture again. In my questioning and overall approach, I had to be especially thorough and tough-minded.

"Are you exercising?" I asked her.

"I run five miles a day, five times a week."

"I want you to stop," I said.

"Are you sure?" She couldn't believe it.

"Positive," I said. "This time, Janet, you must listen to me a hundred percent of the time. Exercise is not getting you anywhere. Exercise is fine, but exercise is perhaps ten to twenty percent of the total picture."

In order for Janet to realize her radical goal, she needed to give herself over to my complete guidance and control. Even though I told Janet we could do this, I truly knew that the task that lay before us was extremely difficult due to the time restraints. I told her, "From now on you must concentrate on your eating and sleeping. It's back to basics. That means you have to destress your body. I need to reset your hunger patterns and reset your metabolism. You need to reheal your body. A new set of diagnostic tests will be helpful in setting a course of action." At this point I had Janet undergo a battery of tests, including extensive blood work to test for blood sugar problems, inflammation, thyroid dysfunction, adrenal issues, liver function, and hormonal imbalances. The results would help me interpret the cumulative effects of her weight gain and elevated stress levels over the previous year.

When it comes to significant weight loss, we need to get our clients to focus on accomplishments step by step. It is imperative that they view the glass as half full, not half empty. Motivation is accelerated by acknowledgment of achievement.

After reviewing the results of Janet's tests we discovered that she had developed dysbiosis of the gastrointestinal (GI) tract, was borderline type 2 diabetic, was suffering from systemic inflammation, was in the latter stages of adrenal fatigue, had elevated cholesterol, and showed signs of poor liver function and secondary hypothyroidism.

I told Janet to stop all exercise at this point. Like most of my clients, she thought I was crazy to suggest this. She wondered how it was possible to lose weight without exercise.

It is a common misconception that intensive fitness and cardio is the most effective method to attain weight loss. Janet has learned firsthand that this is not the case. Her intensive workouts are notorious, as evidenced by her six-pack abs. She is one of the most dedicated and disciplined people I have met. If working out were a surefire way to maintain a healthy weight, Janet Jackson would *never* suffer from weight fluctuations.

But that is simply not the case.

And it is simply not the case for millions of Americans struggling with their own weight issues.

In place of exercise, I put Janet on our 21-Day UltraCleanse program, which is designed around customized supplementation, our exclusive UltraCleanse Plus shake, and a personalized meal plan. All of this was tailored to fit Janet's specific needs.

The next thing that we needed to accomplish was to correct Janet's GI dysfunction, which had developed over the past year. This condition is extremely common with our clients. More than 70 percent of them are dealing with some type of GI problem.

Symptoms of GI tract problems include acid reflux, diarrhea, excessive gas, bloating and gassiness after meals, and nausea.

Most sufferers do not even realize that how they feel is not normal. Some of you may have heard the saying "You are what you eat." This is almost true. But I think the real statement should be "You are what you digest."

For those of you who are embarking on the pursuit of weight loss and good health, you must first address your GI problems in order to be successful.

In the first two weeks on my program, Janet had dropped seven pounds. A week later, she had lost another six pounds and was down to 170. (These results, I must point out, were *without* exercise.)

By the end of January, a month after we'd begun, she hit 162.

It is quite normal for our clients to drop weight very quickly in the beginning, because our detox program is designed to minimize inflammation, and that results in the release of excessive body water. Also, clients are much more focused and motivated during their initial weeks on the program.

By the middle of February, Janet was getting bored with it.

"Those words give me the shivers," I told her.

I knew that meant that she was about to go in a direction that would lead to failure once again. I told her to let me come up with some variations.

"The minute you get bored, you start thinking about reverting back," I told her. "And I know you don't want to go back."

We experience this regularly with our clients. This is why we emphasize a stepping-stone approach. Each phase is a step forward and toward your goal. Now it was time to shepherd Janet into the next phase, which would include introducing new foods and more choices than are allowed in the detox of Phase I.

Janet was moving into Phase II. During this time, I told Janet she could add back in the exercising and dancing. She was having a much harder time, though, with increased cravings and food choices. Once again, she was refocused on work during the day and was less hungry, but then ravenous during the evenings. This was a tricky time for us. We actually needed to increase her caloric and nutrient intake to better match her increased activity.

She hung in there, and by mid-April, Janet was down to 140.

Her goal was to get down to 130 by her fortieth birthday on May 16.

For her (and for most people), this was the part of the journey that seemed the most unyielding. She had come so far, yet she still had a ways to go. The weight loss slows down. But you don't want to measure weight loss in pounds, but rather in percentage of change in your body's composition. The last ten pounds you are striving to lose can be the same percentage of your body composition as the initial twenty-five pounds that you lost. It is vital to continue going forward and not get stuck on a number on a scale.

Janet was kind enough to invite me to her fortieth birthday party. She was dressed in white and looked absolutely radiant. She had done more than achieve her goal of 130 pounds; she had overachieved it! She weighed 120. She'd lost nearly 56 pounds in eighteen weeks. I felt like a proud dad. When she went on *Oprah* to tell her story, she looked more like someone in her twenties than in her forties. It seemed appropriate that her next album was called *20 Y.O.*

At this point, I was so proud of Janet, as I have been seeing thousands of my clients succeed over the past twelve years. I told her we should write a book, because she was so much like all the other people who struggle with their weight, which leads to physical and emotional problems and so much more. People need to know that they can do this.

I'm grateful that Janet had the courage to share her journey.

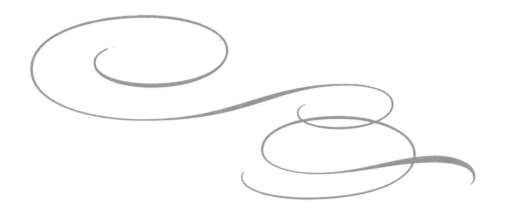

Epilogue

My follow-up album to *20 Y.O.* was called *Discipline*, because I finally realized the absolute necessity for discipline in all aspects of my life—not harsh discipline, but gentle and compassionate discipline, discipline that comes from wanting to move forward rather than fall back into defeat.

David showed me that it takes discipline. Since those dramatic months in 2006, I've continued to fluctuate, but never as drastically or as dangerously as before. Weight remains a challenge. Two steps forward, one step back. I stay in touch with David and keep his principles of balanced nutrition as a part of my life. I do so, however, imperfectly. I still have work to do.

I'll always have work to do—physical as well as emotional. I realized that not everyone has a David Allen and a Tony Martinez or someone to help with food plans. With this book you'll have those tools. I believe we are all capable of activating an inner voice that, to a large degree, duplicates David's.

That voice has some fundamental wisdom to offer that's free to everyone:

Diets don't work. Diets are illusions. Diets are temporary. A plan must be permanent. That requires a change in lifestyle.

The new lifestyle says eat well, eat balanced, eat often. Don't starve yourself. Three good meals. Two healthy snacks.

Exercise is important, but exercise alone is not the answer.

The answer is in proper nutrition.

The answer is in restorative sleep.

The answer is in wholesome foods.

The answer is in self-care—physically, mentally, emotionally, and spiritually.

The answer is within you—the true you.

Recipes

A Note from Chef Andre

I love Janet Jackson. Designing these recipes and cooking for her for *True You* was a dream come true. Janet is a perfectionist and she insisted that everything about these meals be special.

During the weight-loss phase of her program, Janet uses virtually no sodium or sweeteners in these recipes. But these recipes, as presented here, are still low in sodium, sugar, and fat, and are still effective for weight loss and maintenance of a healthy lifestyle.

During weight loss especially, as well as maintenance, please be conscious of portion control. Eat slowly and do not eat beyond the point of hunger. One of Janet's greatest lessons has been to stop eating the moment she feels full. Yes, one extra forkful makes a difference.

And finally, each and every recipe has been tested, tasted, and enjoyed by Janet herself and her friends. These recipes were created especially for *True You*. These recipes were made with love just for you.

Several of the recipes are marked "kid friendly," meaning they were created especially to delight the taste buds of kids and to be enjoyed by the kid in all of us.

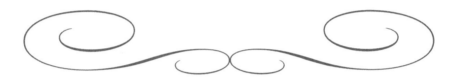

Breakfast

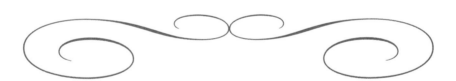

Oatmeal Pancakes (Kid Friendly)

1 cup flour

½ cup quick-cooking oats (not instant)

1 tbsp sugar

½ tsp cinnamon

½ tsp salt

½ tsp baking powder

½ tsp baking soda

1 tbsp canola oil

1 tbsp lemon juice (or vinegar)

about 1¼ cups soy milk

Put 1 tbsp of lemon juice (or vinegar) in a 1-cup measure and fill cup with soy milk. Set aside.

Measure all of the dry ingredients into a bowl and mix together with a spoon.

Pour in the oil, and the soured soy milk. Stir until just mixed. If not thin enough for pancake batter, stir in up to ¼ cup more of soy milk.

Fry in margarine as for regular pancakes.

Serve with fresh sliced strawberries or with maple syrup and margarine.

Makes 5 servings: 2 pancakes each

NUTRITION FACTS

Serving Size 178g

Amount Per Serving

Calories 231

Calories from Fat 53

Daily Value*

Total Fat	5.9g	9%
Saturated Fat	0.6g	3%
Trans Fat	0.0g	
Cholesterol	0mg	0%
Sodium	429mg	18%
Total Carbohydrates	36.3g	12%
Dietary Fiber	2.5g	10%
Sugars	8.1g	
Protein	8.1g	

Vitamin A 0% • Vitamin C 2% • Calcium 7% • Iron 14%

* Based on a 2000 calorie diet

Nutrition Grade B+

Quinoa Breakfast Burrito

1 cup quinoa

2 cups vegetable broth

1 cup cooked red kidney beans

½ cup water

½ tsp minced garlic (I used dried)

½ cup nutritional yeast

Sea salt and freshly ground black pepper, to taste

½ cup water

Sauce:

½ cup salsa

⅛–¼ cup water

1 tbsp nondairy mayonnaise (Vegenaise)

1 tsp cumin

1 tsp pure maple syrup

½ tsp lime juice

¼ tsp chili powder blend

Also:

2 tortillas

avocado, chopped (for garnish)

Add dry, unwashed quinoa to a large dry skillet. Toast until fragrant, stirring occasionally. Add veggie broth and bring to a boil. Cover, lower heat, and simmer until tender (about 15 minutes). Add remaining ingredients (except sauce ingredients), cover, and heat over low heat until beans are warmed through. Add more water if needed to keep the quinoa from sticking.

Sauce: Add all sauce ingredients to a blender and process until sauce is smooth.

In an oven or toaster oven, lightly toast 2 tortillas until warm and slightly crispy. Plate. Divide quinoa/bean mixture in half, and place half the filling inside each tortilla. Roll up or fold tortillas in half.

Serves 4

NUTRITION FACTS

Serving Size 335g   Amount Per Serving

Calories 417   **Calories from Fat 45**

		Daily Value*
Total Fat	5.0g	8%
Saturated Fat	0.7g	4%
Cholesterol	0mg	0%
Sodium	599mg	25%
Total Carbohydrates	68.6g	23%
Dietary Fiber	15.6g	62%
Sugars	3.3g	
Protein	28.6g	

Vitamin A 2% • Vitamin C 5% • Calcium 10% • Iron 54%

* Based on a 2000 calorie diet

Nutrition Grade A

Hot Quinoa Breakfast Cereal

Quinoa has a unique, nutty taste and cooks in just 12 minutes.
A gluten-free whole grain, rich in dietary fiber, providing 45 percent
daily value (DV). Best amino acid profile of all cereal grains.

---

1 cup quinoa

2 cups water

½ cup apples, thinly sliced

⅓ cup raisins

½ tsp cinnamon

Soy milk or almond milk

Sweeten with agave, honey, maple syrup, brown sugar, or sweetener
   of choice

Rinse quinoa and add to water; bring to a boil. Reduce heat; simmer for 5 minutes. Add apples, raisins, and cinnamon; simmer until water is absorbed. Serve with soy milk or almond milk and sweeten to taste.

Serve hot. Garnish with toasted almonds

Serves 4

NUTRITION FACTS

Serving Size 187g	Amount Per Serving	
Calories 200	**Calories from Fat 24**	
		Daily Value*
Total Fat	2.7g	4%
Trans Fat	0.0g	
Cholesterol	0mg	0%
Sodium	7mg	0%
Total Carbohydrates	39.0g	13%
Dietary Fiber	3.9g	16%
Sugars	8.6g	
Protein	6.4g	

Vitamin A 0% • Vitamin C 2% • Calcium 3% • Iron 12%

Janet Jackson

* Based on a 2000 calorie diet

Nutrition Grade A

Veggie Baked Eggs

2 tbsp sweet onion, thinly sliced

4 mushrooms, thinly sliced

2 tbsp chopped red bell pepper

1 tsp thyme

¼ tsp paprika

¼ tsp garlic powder

4 tbsp parmesan cheese or a low-fat cheese of choice

4 eggs

salt

pepper

Italian parsley, chopped

Cooking spray—butter flavor

Preheat oven to 325°F.

Spray 4 muffin tins or small oven-proof dishes with cooking spray.

Combine veggies and season with thyme, paprika, and garlic powder.

194

Place equal amounts of vegetables in each tin, top each one with 1 tbsp of the cheese.

Break egg into each dish. Sprinkle lightly with salt and pepper.

Bake, uncovered, until eggs are set to your liking (15–18 minutes).

Sprinkle with parsley before serving.

Serves 4

NUTRITION FACTS

Serving Size 77g

Amount Per Serving

Calories 94

Calories from Fat 53

		Daily Value*
Total Fat	5.9g	9%
Saturated Fat	2.2g	11%
Cholesterol	191mg	64%
Sodium	140mg	6%
Total Carbohydrates	2.2g	1%
Dietary Fiber	0.5g	2%
Sugars	1.2g	
Protein	8.2g	

Vitamin A 9% • Vitamin C 12% • Calcium 9% • Iron 7%

* Based on a 2000 calorie diet

Nutrition Grade A

Whole-Wheat Fruity Breakfast Bars

Loaded with fruits and whole grain, this is great for breakfast on the go.

2 cups organic wheat flour

1½ cups oats, toasted

1 tsp ground cinnamon

¼ tsp salt

½ cup butter

½ cup brown sugar or sweetener

½ cup honey

2 ripe bananas, mashed

1 apple, peeled, cored, and diced

1 cup blueberries

1 cup dried cranberries

1 tbsp orange zest

1 cup orange juice

Preheat oven to 350°F.

In medium bowl add the flour, toasted oats, cinnamon, and salt. Mix well.

In your stand mixer (or handheld) with paddle attachment, cream the butter and the sugar until they're fluffy. About 5–8 minutes at medium speed.

In the meantime, in a separate bowl, mash the bananas, with honey, add the rest of the fruit to combine.

Add the flour slowly to the sugar-butter mixture. Mix on low.

Then add the orange juice and zest. Mix briefly, just until everything is incorporated. Gently fold in fruits using spatula.

Coat a 9x13-inch baking dish with vegetable spray and spread dough evenly. Bake 25–30 minutes or until toothpick inserted in center comes out clean.

Makes about 12 bars

Great for lunch boxes, too!

NUTRITION FACTS

Serving Size 133g

Calories 293

	Amount Per Serving	
	Calories from Fat 78	
		Daily Value*
Total Fat	8.7g	13%
Saturated Fat	5.0g	25%
Trans Fat	0.0g	
Cholesterol	20mg	7%
Sodium	109mg	5%
Total Carbohydrates	51.6g	17%
Dietary Fiber	3.3g	13%
Sugars	24.5g	
Protein	4.1g	

Vitamin A 6%　•　Vitamin C 26%　•　Calcium 2%　•　Iron 9%

* Based on a 2000 calorie diet

Nutrition Grade B

All-In-One Smoothie

1 banana

1 cup berries, blueberries and/or strawberries, fresh or frozen

1 cup orange juice, preferably calcium-fortified

½ cup soy milk or almond milk

2 tbsp raw almonds, or almond butter

1 tbsp honey or sweetener

1 cup of ice

Combine all ingredients in a blender; cover and blend until creamy. Serve immediately.

It might be a little weird to drink chopped almonds but they will add a nice texture to your smoothie.

Serves 2

NUTRITION FACTS

Serving Size 389g   Amount Per Serving

Calories 275   **Calories from Fat 99**

		Daily Value*
Total Fat	11.0g	17%
Saturated Fat	1.1g	6%
Trans Fat	0.0g	
Cholesterol	0mg	0%
Sodium	39mg	2%
Total Carbohydrates	42.3g	14%
Dietary Fiber	2.8g	11%

True You

Sugars	28.7g
Protein	6.0g

Vitamin A 6% • Vitamin C 112% • Calcium 8% • Iron 8%

* Based on a 2000 calorie diet

Nutrition Grade B+

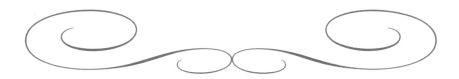

Lunch/Dinner

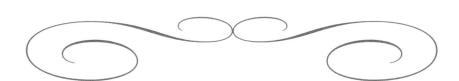

Baked Ziti (Kid Friendly)

1 pound dry ziti pasta

2 tbsp olive oil

1 onion, chopped

1 pound ground turkey

1 tsp ground cumin

1 tsp garlic powder

½ tsp pepper flakes

8 oz raw spinach

2 (26 oz) jars spaghetti sauce—low sodium

6 oz provolone cheese, sliced

1½ cups light sour cream

6 oz mozzarella cheese, shredded

2 tbsp Parmesan cheese, grated

Bring a large pot of lightly salted water to a boil. Add ziti pasta and cook until al dente, about 8 minutes; drain.

In a large skillet with olive oil, brown onion and ground turkey over medium heat. Season with cumin, garlic, and pepper flakes; add spinach, cook for 5 minutes, then add spaghetti sauce, and simmer for 15 minutes.

Preheat the oven to 350°F.

Spray a 9x13-inch baking dish with cooking spray. Layer as follows: half of the ziti, Provolone cheese, sour cream, half of the meat/sauce mixture, remaining ziti, mozzarella cheese, and remaining meat/sauce mixture. Top with grated Parmesan cheese.

Bake for 30 minutes in the preheated oven, or until cheeses are melted.

Serves 5–6

NUTRITION FACTS

Serving Size 517g

Amount Per Serving

Calories 1,337

Calories from Fat 293

Daily Value*

Total Fat	32.6g	50%
Saturated Fat	13.8g	69%
Cholesterol	169mg	56%
Sodium	169mg	7%
Total Carbohydrates	204.6g	68%
Dietary Fiber	8.6g	34%
Sugars	1.4g	
Protein	60.6g	

Vitamin A 80% • Vitamin C 28% • Calcium 94% • Iron 67%

* Based on a 2000 calorie diet

Nutrition Grade B

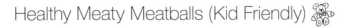

Healthy Meaty Meatballs (Kid Friendly)

1 lb ground turkey

1 lb ground turkey sausage (can be spicy for extra kick)

2 eggs

3 cloves garlic, finely chopped

¼ cup fresh parsley, chopped

¼ cup Parmesan cheese, grated

1 cup soft bread crumbs

2 tbsp milk

1 tbsp olive oil

salt and ground black pepper

In a large mixing bowl, combine all ingredients, mix well. Shape into 16 balls of equal size.

Heat the oil in a skillet large enough to hold the meatballs in one layer without touching. Cook until nicely browned all over, at least 10 minutes.

Drain the meatballs and place them in a saucepan with marinara sauce. Simmer 25–30 minutes, depending on the amount and what marinara sauce you are using, stirring occasionally. If doing a homemade sauce, simmer 50–60 minutes.

About 10 minutes before the meatballs have finished cooking, cook spaghetti as directed on package. Drain well.

Serve the meatballs and sauce on the spaghetti, sprinkled with extra Parmesan cheese.

You can skip step 2 and place meatballs right into simmering marinara sauce, 45–50 minutes. Your meatballs won't have a nice brown color but they will be just as tasty.

Serves 4 people, 4 meatballs each

NUTRITION FACTS

Serving Size 167g

Calories 387

Amount Per Serving

Calories from Fat 205

		Daily Value*
Total Fat	22.8g	35%
Saturated Fat	6.2g	31%
Cholesterol	215mg	72%
Sodium	313mg	13%
Total Carbohydrates	6.2g	2%
Sugars	1.1g	
Protein	37.4g	

Vitamin A 9% • Vitamin C 10% • Calcium 14% • Iron 18%

* Based on a 2000 calorie diet

Nutrition Grade B+

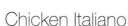

Chicken Italiano

2 tbsp olive oil

½ cup chopped sweet onion

2 cloves garlic, minced

1 tsp fresh oregano

½ cup sun-dried tomatoes, chopped

1 cup chicken broth

1 pound skinless, boneless chicken breast halves (about 5 breasts)

salt and pepper

2 tbsp vegetable oil

2 tbsp chopped fresh basil

In a large saucepan over medium heat, add olive oil, onion, and garlic, cook for about 1 minute.

Add the tomatoes, oregano, and chicken broth; bring to a boil. Reduce heat and simmer, uncovered, for about 10 minutes or until the tomatoes are tender. While this is simmering, season chicken with salt and pepper on both sides.

In a large skillet over medium heat, warm vegetable oil and sauté chicken. Cook for about 4 minutes per side or until meat is no longer pink inside. Transfer chicken to first skillet and add fresh basil. Cover chicken with broth mixture and serve.

Serves 4–6

NUTRITION FACTS

Serving Size 149g	Amount Per Serving	
Calories 169	Calories from Fat 99	
		Daily Value*
Total Fat	11.0g	17%
Saturated Fat	1.9g	10%
Cholesterol	44mg	15%
Sodium	250mg	10%
Total Carbohydrates	2.0g	1%
Sugars	0.9g	
Protein	16.7g	

Vitamin A 3% • Vitamin C 5% • Calcium 1% • Iron 2%

* Based on a 2000 calorie diet

Nutrition Grade D+

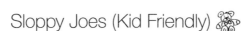

Sloppy Joes (Kid Friendly)

For healthy, lean, and mean sloppy joes we start with lean ground turkey and top them off with 100 percent whole-wheat buns.

1 pound lean ground turkey

1 cup chopped onion

1 cup chopped green bell pepper

1 tbsp brown sugar

1 tsp ground cumin

1 tbsp apple cider vinegar

1 cup ketchup

2 tbsp tomato paste

2 tbsp prepared mustard

1 tsp ground cloves

1 tsp salt

4 whole-wheat hamburger buns

In a large skillet over medium heat, combine the ground turkey, onion, and green pepper. Cook until meat is browned, breaking up the meat into crumbles as it cooks, then drain off excess drippings.

Stir in the brown sugar, cumin, vinegar, ketchup, tomato paste, and mustard, and season with cloves and salt.

Simmer for 30 minutes on low.

Place a scoop of the mixture onto each bun and serve.

Serves 4

NUTRITION FACTS

Serving Size 249g   Amount Per Serving

Calories 262   **Calories from Fat 80**

		Daily Value*
Total Fat	8.9g	14%
Saturated Fat	2.6g	13%
Trans Fat	0.0g	
Cholesterol	81mg	27%
Sodium	1436mg	60%
Total Carbohydrates	23.6g	8%
Dietary Fiber	1.8g	7%
Sugars	19.1g	
Protein	24.6g	

Vitamin A 28% • Vitamin C 71% • Calcium 3% • Iron 7%

* Based on a 2000 calorie diet

Nutrition Grade B

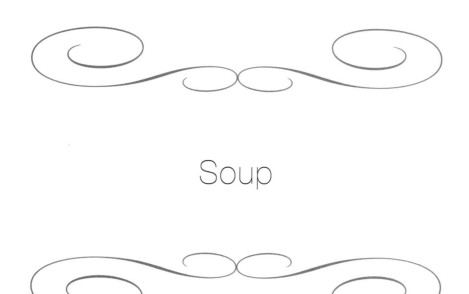

Soup

Carrot, Yam, and Rosemary Soup

1 small onion, chopped

1 tbsp vegetable oil

5 medium carrots, chopped

1 small yam, peeled and chopped

4 cups vegetable stock

3 sprigs of rosemary

2 tbsp lemon juice

Salt and ground pepper

Soften onions in a large pan with oil. Add the chopped carrots, yam, stock, whole springs of rosemary, and lemon juice.

Bring to a boil, cover and cook for 20 minutes.

When carrots and yam are very tender remove rosemary, puree the soup in a blender or food processor (you may need to do this in halves), return soup to pan, and season to taste.

Heat through again, serve with a wonderful warm whole-grain bread.

Serves 4–6

NUTRITION FACTS

Serving Size 105g   Amount Per Serving

Calories 70   **Calories from Fat 32**

		Daily Value*
Total Fat	3.6g	6%
Saturated Fat	0.7g	4%
Trans Fat	0.0g	
Cholesterol	0mg	0%
Sodium	53mg	2%
Total Carbohydrates	9.6g	3%
Dietary Fiber	2.5g	10%
Sugars	4.5g	
Protein	0.9g	

Vitamin A 255%   •   Vitamin C 16%   •   Calcium 3%   •   Iron 2%

* Based on a 2000 calorie diet

Nutrition Grade A

Zesty Red Bell Pepper Soup

4 red bell peppers, seeded and chopped

1 large onion, chopped

4 tbsp olive oil

2 garlic cloves, crushed

3 tbsp tomato paste

3½ cups vegetable stock

2 tsp dried cilantro

1 tsp smoked paprika

salt and ground black pepper

cilantro leaves to garnish

In a large saucepan, cook peppers and onion gently in the oil for about 5 minutes, stirring occasionally.

Stir in the garlic, dried cilantro, paprika, and tomato paste. Add in half the stock, bring to a boil.

Cover the pan, lower the heat, and simmer for 10 minutes.

Puree the mixture in a food processor or blender. Return to the pan; add the remaining stock for desired consistency, season with salt and pepper.

Bring soup back to a boil, allow to heat through.

Garnish with cilantro leaves.

Serves 4

NUTRITION FACTS

Serving Size 184g

Calories 185

Amount Per Serving

Calories from Fat 126

		Daily Value*
Total Fat	14.0g	22%
Saturated Fat	1.9g	10%
Cholesterol	0mg	0%
Sodium	19mg	1%
Total Carbohydrates	13.8g	5%
Dietary Fiber	3.9g	15%
Sugars	8.1g	
Protein	2.3g	

Vitamin A 84%　•　Vitamin C 264%　•　Calcium 3%　•　Iron 7%

* Based on a 2000 calorie diet

Nutrition Grade B+

⌒

White Bean Soup with White Truffle Oil

Warm and delicious on a cool autumn night

1 cup sliced carrots

½ cup chopped onion

1 clove garlic, minced

1 tbsp olive oil

2 cans (15 oz each) white kidney beans, rinsed and drained

2 cans (14½ oz each) vegetable broth or chicken both

½ tsp dried oregano, crushed

¼ tsp fresh ground pepper

⅛ tsp chipotle pepper

2 tbsp white truffle oil

Plum tomato halves, if desired

Chopped fresh parsley, if desired

In a large saucepan over medium heat, sauté carrots, onion, and garlic for 5 minutes or until onion is tender, stirring occasionally. Add beans, broth, and seasonings (not truffle oil). Bring to a boil. Reduce heat; cover and simmer 10 minutes.

To serve, ladle into individual serving bowls. Garnish with tomatoes and parsley and drizzle with truffle oil.

Serves 6

NUTRITION FACTS

Serving Size 8 oz

	Amount Per Serving	
Calories 64	Calories from Fat 31	
		Daily Value*
Total Fat	3.4g	5%
Saturated Fat	0.6g	3%
Trans Fat	0.0g	
Cholesterol	0mg	0%
Sodium	642mg	27%
Total Carbohydrates	3.7g	1%
Dietary Fiber	0.8g	3%
Sugars	1.9g	
Protein	4.3g	

Vitamin A 61% • Vitamin C 4% • Calcium 2% • Iron 3%

* Based on a 2000 calorie diet

Nutrition Grade B+

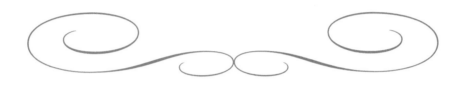

Salad

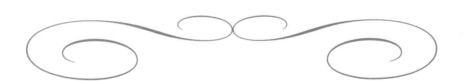

Avocado, Black Bean, and Corn Salad (ABC Salad)

1 (15 oz) can of black beans, thoroughly rinsed and drained (or
    1½ cups freshly cooked black beans)

1½ cups roasted corn, can be frozen, allow to come to room
    temperature

½ cup chopped green onions

3 fresh plum tomatoes, seeded and chopped

2 avocados, peeled, seeded, and cut into chunks

½ cup fresh chopped cilantro

½ tsp garlic powder

½ tsp cumin powder

2 tbsp lime juice (about the juice from one lime)

1 tbsp olive oil

Salt and pepper to taste

Make sure to rinse and drain beans well.

In a large bowl, combine the beans, corn, onions, tomatoes, avocado, cilantro, garlic powder, cumin, lime juice, and olive oil. Salt and pepper to taste.

Chill before serving.

Serves 6–8

NUTRITION FACTS

Serving Size 217g

Amount Per Serving

Calories 389

Calories from Fat 119

		Daily Value*
Total Fat	13.3g	20%
Saturated Fat	2.0g	10%
Cholesterol	0mg	0%
Sodium	19mg	1%
Total Carbohydrates	54.4g	18%
Dietary Fiber	16.3g	65%
Sugars	4.8g	
Protein	17.7g	

Vitamin A 13% • Vitamin C 41% • Calcium 11% • Iron 25%

* Based on a 2000 calorie diet

Nutrition Grade A

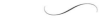

Mixed Baby Greens with Fresh Mango and Raspberry Honey Vinaigrette

4 cups mixed lettuce greens

1 large mango, peeled and cut into chunks

1 tbsp raspberry preserves, seedless

1 tbsp honey

1 tsp Dijon mustard

1 garlic clove, minced

2 tbsp green onion, chopped

¼ cup balsamic vinegar

3 tbsp extra-virgin olive oil

½ tsp chopped fresh mint

Salt and pepper to taste

Combine raspberry preserves, honey, mustard, and garlic in small bowl; mix well. Add green onion, vinegar, olive oil, mint, and salt and pepper to taste. Blend well.

To serve, combine greens with mango, drizzle half the raspberry honey vinaigrette over lettuce greens. Toss to coat.

Use remaining vinaigrette as needed.

NUTRITION FACTS

Serving Size 3 oz

Amount Per Serving

Calories 133 Calories from Fat 92

		Daily Value*
Total Fat	10.3g	16%
Saturated Fat	1.4g	7%
Trans Fat	0.0g	
Cholesterol	0mg	0%
Sodium	23mg	1%
Total Carbohydrates	10.1g	3%
Dietary Fiber	0.9g	4%
Sugars	8.0g	
Protein	0.7g	

Vitamin A 6% • Vitamin C 5% • Calcium 2% • Iron 3%

* Based on a 2000 calorie diet

Nutrition Grade C

Strawberry Spinach Salad

1 cup fresh strawberries, sliced
bunch of spinach, washed thoroughly
3 tbsp balsamic vinegar

In a bowl, place strawberries and balsamic vinegar, allow to marinate for about 15 minutes.

Wash spinach thoroughly.

Drain the vinegar from the strawberries and use this vinegar to make your vinaigrette.

Toss the strawberries and spinach and the vinaigrette and serve.

Strawberry Balsamic Vinaigrette:
2 tbsp olive oil
3 tbsp balsamic vinegar (from the strawberries)
¼ tsp crushed garlic
¼ tsp dried oregano
salt and pepper to taste

Save a little dressing for another day.

Serves 2

NUTRITION FACTS

Serving Size 301g

Amount Per Serving

Calories 192

Calories from Fat 130

		Daily Value*
Total Fat	14.4g	22%
Saturated Fat	2.0g	10%
Trans Fat	0.0g	
Cholesterol	0mg	0%
Sodium	138mg	6%
Total Carbohydrates	12.2g	4%
Dietary Fiber	5.3g	21%
Sugars	4.4g	
Protein	5.4g	

Vitamin A 319% • Vitamin C 150% • Calcium 19% • Iron 29%

* Based on a 2000 calorie diet

Nutrition Grade A

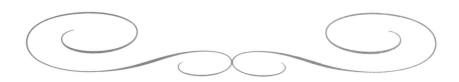

Starters & Sides

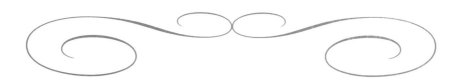

Chipotle Roasted Sweet Potatoes with Cilantro

4 large sweet potatoes, peeled and cut into bite-sized chunks

1 medium sweet onion, peeled and chopped

2 tbsp olive oil

salt

freshly ground pepper

chipotle powder

cooking spray

2 tbsp minced fresh cilantro

Position rack in bottom third of oven and preheat to 400°F.

Toss sweet potatoes and onion with olive oil, salt and pepper, and just a dash of chipotle powder (go lightly, you can always add more later) in large bowl to coat.

Spray baking sheet generously with cooking spray. Spread sweet potatoes and onion in a single layer on baking sheet.

Roast until tender and golden brown, stirring occasionally, about 20–25 minutes.

Transfer to serving bowl and sprinkle with cilantro.

Serves 8

NUTRITION FACTS

Serving Size 18g   Amount Per Serving

Calories 36   **Calories from Fat 31**

		Daily Value*
Total Fat	3.5g	5%
Trans Fat	0.0g	
Cholesterol	0mg	0%
Sodium	20mg	1%
Total Carbohydrates	1.3g	0%
Sugars	0.6g	
Protein	0.2g	

Vitamin A 0%   •   Vitamin C 2%   •   Calcium 0%   •   Iron 0%

* Based on a 2000 calorie diet

Nutrition Grade C

Baked Oven Fries (Kid Friendly)

3 russet potatoes (about 24 oz total), peeled and cut lengthwise into
    even-sized wedges

5 tbsp vegetable, canola, or peanut oil, divided

¾ tsp kosher salt, plus more to taste

¼ tsp freshly ground black pepper, plus more to taste

1 tbsp chopped cilantro or Italian parsley for garnish

Preheat the oven to 475°F.

Place the potato wedges in a large mixing bowl. Cover with hot water; soak for 10–30 minutes. Put 4 tablespoons of the oil onto a heavy rimmed baking sheet. Tilt the sheet from side to side to evenly coat the pan with oil (a pastry brush can also help with this). Sprinkle the pan evenly with the salt and pepper. Set aside.

Drain the potatoes. Spread the wedges out on layers of paper towels or on clean kitchen towels. Pat dry with additional towels. Wipe out the now empty bowl so it is dry. Return the potatoes to the bowl and toss with the remaining 1 tablespoon of oil. Arrange the potato wedges on the prepared baking sheet in a single layer. Cover tightly with foil and bake for 5 minutes.

Remove the foil and continue to bake until the bottoms of the potatoes are spotty golden brown, 15–20 minutes, rotating the baking sheet after 10 minutes. Using a metal spatula and tongs, flip each potato wedge, keeping them in a single layer.

Continue baking until the fries are golden and crisp, 5–15 minutes. Rotate the pan as needed to ensure even browning.

When the fries are finished baking, transfer to a paper-towel-lined plate to drain some of the grease. Season with additional salt and pepper to taste. Garnish with chopped cilantro or parsley.

Serve warm.

NUTRITION FACTS

Serving Size 179g	Amount Per Serving	
Calories 260	**Calories from Fat 153**	
		Daily Value*
Total Fat	17.1g	26%
Saturated Fat	2.9g	14%

Cholesterol	0mg	0%
Sodium	448mg	19%
Total Carbohydrates	25.2g	8%
Dietary Fiber	3.9g	16%
Sugars	1.9g	
Protein	2.7g	

Vitamin A 2% • Vitamin C 55% • Calcium 2% • Iron 5%

* Based on a 2000 calorie diet

Nutrition Grade B

Grilled Asparagus with Cilantro-Lime Dressing

1½ to 2 lbs large asparagus

2 tbsp olive oil

salt and pepper

juice of 3 limes

2 tbsp shallots, minced

¼ cup fresh cilantro, minced

Snap off the woody ends of the asparagus; most spears will break naturally an inch or two above the bottom. Meanwhile, start a charcoal fire or preheat a gas grill

Asparagus: toss them with about 1 tbsp of the oil, mixing with your hands until they're coated. Season well with salt and pepper to taste. Grill until tender and browned in spots, turning once or twice, a total of 5 to 10 minutes.

To pan-grill the asparagus, do not oil or season them. Just toss them in the hot skillet and cook, turning the individual spears as they brown, until tender, 5 to 10 minutes. Remove as they finish, and season with salt and pepper.

Mix together the lime juice and shallots, then stir in enough olive oil to add a little body; the mixture should still be quite strong. Season it with salt and pepper and stir in the cilantro. Serve the asparagus hot or at room temperature.

Serves 4

NUTRITION FACTS

Serving Size 255g	Amount Per Serving	
Calories 113	Calories from Fat 63	
		Daily Value*
Total Fat	7.0g	11%
Saturated Fat	1.0g	5%
Cholesterol	0mg	0%
Sodium	6mg	0%
Total Carbohydrates	11.0g	4%
Dietary Fiber	4.9g	19%
Sugars	4.5g	
Protein	5.2g	

Vitamin A 37% • Vitamin C 30% • Calcium 6% • Iron 28%

* Based on a 2000 calorie diet

Nutrition Grade A

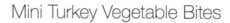

Mini Turkey Vegetable Bites

1 cup whole-wheat bread crumbs

1 tbsp olive oil

½ cup sweet onion, diced

½ cup zucchini, diced

½ cup red pepper, diced

½ cup sliced fresh mushrooms

1 lb ground turkey

1 large egg

½ tsp salt

¼ tsp freshly ground black pepper

Preheat oven to 350°F.

Spray muffin tin with nonstick cooking spray.

Combine all ingredients well and fill muffin cups with meat mixture. Bake 20 to 30 minutes until set and browned on top.

Serve hot or at room temperature.

Makes 12 mini bites

NUTRITION FACTS

Serving Size 119g	Amount Per Serving	
Calories 219	**Calories from Fat 118**	
		Daily Value*
Total Fat	13.1g	20%
Saturated Fat	3.1g	16%

Cholesterol	112mg	37%
Sodium	288mg	12%
Total Carbohydrates	2.0g	1%
Dietary Fiber	0.5g	2%
Sugars	1.0g	
Protein	22.2g	

Vitamin A 6% • Vitamin C 20% • Calcium 3% • Iron 10%

* Based on a 2000 calorie diet

Nutrition Grade B

Roasted Corn, Cherry Tomatoes with Sweet Peas and Basil

2 tbsp olive oil

2 cups sweet corn kernels (about 2 large ears, fresh corn)

1½ cups fresh sweet peas or frozen, thawed

2 cups cherry tomatoes, halved

¾ cup toasted pine nuts

¼ cup julienned basil leaves

pinch of chipotle powder

2 tbsp olive oil

salt and pepper to taste

In a large nonstick skillet set over medium-high heat, heat 2 tbsp oil until hot. Add corn and sauté until just cooked, about 3 minutes. Transfer to a bowl and let cool. Add peas, tomatoes, another 2 tbsp olive oil, chipotle powder, basil and pine nuts. Drizzle with a little olive oil, season with salt and fresh ground pepper to taste.

Serve at room temperature.

Serves 4

NUTRITION FACTS

Serving Size 111g	Amount Per Serving	
Calories 275	Calories from Fat 224	
		Daily Value*
Total Fat	24.9g	38%
Saturated Fat	4.9g	24%
Cholesterol	0mg	0%
Sodium	4mg	0%
Total Carbohydrates	9.7g	3%
Dietary Fiber	3.9g	16%
Sugars	2.7g	
Protein	3.7g	

Vitamin A 12% • Vitamin C 17% • Calcium 1% • Iron 6%

* Based on a 2000 calorie diet

Nutrition Grade C

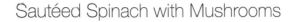

Sautéed Spinach with Mushrooms

1 lb fresh spinach

3 tbsp extra virgin olive oil

½ lb mushrooms, thickly sliced

salt and pepper

½ tbsp finely chopped garlic

pinch of red pepper flakes

Wash and drain spinach very well. Use a salad spinner or dry in a colander.

Heat 2 tbsp olive oil in a skillet. Add the mushrooms and salt and pepper to taste. Cook, stirring often, over high heat until the mushrooms are browned.

Add garlic and remaining oil, spinach and pepper flakes. Cook, stirring, about 30 seconds. Serve hot.

Serves 4

NUTRITION FACTS

Serving Size 181g	Amount Per Serving	
Calories 130	Calories from Fat 97	
		Daily Value*
Total Fat	10.8g	17%
Saturated Fat	1.5g	7%
Cholesterol	0mg	0%
Sodium	93mg	4%

Total Carbohydrates	6.4g	2%
Dietary Fiber	3.1g	12%
Sugars	1.4g	
Protein	5.1g	

Vitamin A 213% • Vitamin C 56% • Calcium 12% • Iron 19%

* Based on a 2000 calorie diet

Nutrition Grade A

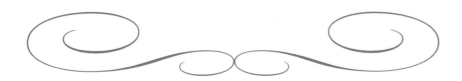

Snacks

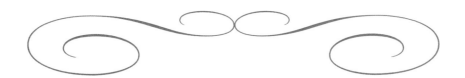

Cauliflower Popcorn

4-inch segment of a thin day-old baguette
1 medium head of cauliflower, washed
extra-virgin olive oil
½ teaspoon salt

Preheat oven to 400°F and place racks in the middle.

Place baguette in a food processor until you have textured, not-too-fine bread crumbs.

Trim the cauliflower. Get rid of the big stalks and stems and strive for uniform, bite-sized little florets.

In a big bowl toss the cauliflower with a few generous table-spoons of olive oil and the salt. Toss until the cauliflower is well coated and then place it in a single layer on a rimmed baking sheet. You are going to bake for about 25–30 minutes total.

There will be some residual olive oil in the big bowl you used to toss the cauliflower. If not, add another tablespoon or two. Add the bread crumbs, mix.

After the cauliflower has been baking for about 15–20 minutes anything in contact with the pan should be nicely browned. Pull the pan out of the oven, rotate each piece of cauliflower so that another side will get some color, and then sprinkle the entire pan with the bread crumb mixture. Return the pan to the oven and finish with another 10 minutes or so. The cauliflower should be tender throughout and the bread crumbs nicely toasted. Serve immediately; it really isn't half as delicious after it has been sitting on the counter getting cold.

Serves 4

NUTRITION FACTS

Serving Size 208g

Amount Per Serving

Calories 90 — Calories from Fat 42

		Daily Value*
Total Fat	4.7g	7%
Saturated Fat	0.7g	3%
Cholesterol	0mg	0%
Sodium	1223mg	51%
Total Carbohydrates	10.6g	4%
Dietary Fiber	5.0g	20%
Sugars	4.8g	
Protein	4.0g	

Vitamin A 1%   •   Vitamin C 155%   •   Calcium 4%   •   Iron 5%

* Based on a 2000 calorie diet

Nutrition Grade A

Crispy Baked Veggies (Kid Friendly)

2 cups fresh veggies (carrots, zucchini, red or green sweet pepper,
broccoli or cauliflower)

1 egg

¼ cup 2% low-fat milk

1 tbsp canola oil

Dry Mixture

2 cups Japanese bread crumbs (panko)

¼ cup Parmesan cheese

¼ tsp black pepper

¼ tsp salt

½ tsp garlic powder

2 tbsp Parmesan cheese for garnish

Preheat oven to 450°F. Spray cookie sheet with nonstick cooking oil.

Cut carrot, zucchini, and sweet pepper into ¼-inch strips. Chop broccoli and cauliflower into florets.

Beat egg, milk, and oil with a fork in a shallow dish. Combine dry mixture ingredients in a bag; shake well and place in a separate dish.

Dip vegetables into egg mixture, then into breading mixture. Make sure to coat well.

Place on cookie sheet.

Repeat step until all vegetables are coated. Bake 5 minutes.

Remove pan from oven and turn vegetables over with tongs or spatula. Return vegetables to oven and bake for another 5 minutes until vegetables are crisp and tender and the coating is golden brown.

Remove and sprinkle with remaining Parmesan cheese.

NUTRITION FACTS

Serving Size 2 oz

Amount Per Serving

Calories 56 Calories from Fat 39

		% Daily Value*
Total Fat	4.3g	7%
Saturated Fat	1.1g	6%
Trans Fat	0.0g	
Cholesterol	35mg	12%
Sodium	175mg	7%
Total Carbohydrates	1.7g	1%
Sugars	0.8g	
Protein	3.0g	

Vitamin A 3%   •   Vitamin C 11%   •   Calcium 6%   •   Iron 2%

* Based on a 2000 calorie diet

Nutrition Grade B

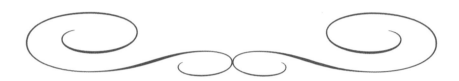

Dessert

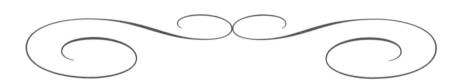

Berries in Balsamic Vinegar with Vanilla and Honey

¼ cup balsamic vinegar

2 tbsp honey

1 tsp vanilla extract

½ cup sliced strawberries

½ cup blueberries

2 walnut orange shortbreads (see recipe)

fresh mint

In a small bowl, whisk together the balsamic vinegar, honey, and vanilla.

In another bowl, add the strawberries and blueberries. Pour the balsamic vinegar mixture over the berries. Let the fruit marinate for 10 to 15 minutes.

Drain the marinade. Refrigerate or serve immediately.

To serve, divide the berries into 2 serving dishes, with short-bread on the side. Garnish with fresh mint.

Serves 2

NUTRITION FACTS

Serving Size 125g

Calories 108

Amount Per Serving

Calories from Fat 2

Janet Jackson

		Daily Value*
Total Fat	0.2g	0%
Trans Fat	0.0g	
Cholesterol	0mg	0%
Sodium	3mg	0%
Total Carbohydrates	25.9g	9%
Dietary Fiber	1.6g	7%
Sugars	23.0g	
Protein	0.6g	

Vitamin A 0% • Vitamin C 41% • Calcium 1% • Iron 2%

* Based on a 2000 calorie diet

Nutrition Grade B

Blueberry Peach Crumble

8 ripe peaches, peeled, pitted, and sliced

½ cup fresh blueberries

Juice from 1 lemon

⅓ tsp ground cinnamon

¼ tsp ground nutmeg

½ cup whole-wheat flour

¼ cup packed dark brown sugar

2 tbsp trans-fat-free margarine, cut into thin slices

¼ cup quick-cooking oats

2 tbsp finely chopped almonds

Preheat the oven to 375°F.

Lightly coat an 8x8-inch baking dish with cooking spray.

In a medium bowl gently combine peach slices, blueberries, lemon juice, cinnamon, and nutmeg. Transfer to baking dish.

In a small bowl, whisk together flour and brown sugar. With your fingers, crumble the margarine into the flour-sugar mixture. Add the oats and almonds, mix evenly. Sprinkle the flour mixture on top of the fruit.

Bake until peaches are soft and the topping is browned, about 30 minutes. Remove from oven and serve warm.

Serves 8

NUTRITION FACTS

Serving Size 119g

Amount Per Serving

Calories 91   **Calories from Fat 12**

Daily Value*

Total Fat	1.3g	2%
Trans Fat	0.0g	
Cholesterol	0mg	0%
Sodium	0mg	0%
Total Carbohydrates	18.8g	6%
Dietary Fiber	2.4g	10%
Sugars	9.2g	
Protein	2.4g	

Vitamin A 6% • Vitamin C 12% • Calcium 1% • Iron 5%

* Based on a 2000 calorie diet

Nutrition Grade A

Chocolate Pudding

½ cup brown sugar

3 tbsp unsweetened cocoa powder

¼ cup cornstarch

⅛ tsp salt

2½ cups low-fat milk

2 tbsp margarine or butter

3 tbsp chocolate chips

1 tsp vanilla extract

In a medium saucepan combine brown sugar, cocoa, cornstarch, salt, and milk. Over medium heat whisk constantly, until the mixture comes to a boil and bubbles and thickens. Remove from heat.

Add chocolate chips and vanilla; stir until the chips have melted.

Let cool briefly, serve warm, or transfer to a bowl, refrigerate until chilled and ready to serve.

Serves 4–6

NUTRITION FACTS

Serving Size 100g

Calories 269

Amount Per Serving

Calories from Fat 90

		Daily Value*
Total Fat	10.1g	15%
Saturated Fat	3.9g	19%
Cholesterol	9mg	3%
Sodium	220mg	9%
Total Carbohydrates	39.8g	13%
Dietary Fiber	1.7g	7%
Sugars	29.8g	
Protein	6.6g	

Vitamin A 11% • Vitamin C 0% • Calcium 22% • Iron 5%

* Based on a 2000 calorie diet

Nutrition Grade C

Fresh Fruit Kebabs with Honey Yogurt Coconut Dip

32 oz Greek honey yogurt

2 tbsp orange blossom honey

½ tsp lime zest

¼ cup coconut flakes, lightly toasted

16 pineapple chunks

8 strawberries, halved

2 kiwi, peeled and diced

2 mangoes, peeled and cut into chunks

2 bananas, cut into ½-inch chunks

8 red grapes

8 wooden skewers

In a small bowl, whisk together the yogurt, honey, and lime zest. Cover and refrigerate until needed.

Alternating, thread fruit onto each skewer, placing a grape on last. Just before serving, fold in toasted coconut flakes into honey yogurt dip and serve.

Serves 4

NUTRITION FACTS

Serving Size 240g

Amount Per Serving

Calories 200

Calories from Fat 22

		Daily Value*
Total Fat	2.4g	4%
Saturated Fat	1.6g	8%
Cholesterol	0mg	0%
Sodium	5mg	0%
Total Carbohydrates	47.9g	16%
Dietary Fiber	5.5g	22%
Sugars	36.1g	
Protein	2.0g	

Vitamin A 17%   •   Vitamin C 139%   •   Calcium 3%   •   Iron 4%

* Based on a 2000 calorie diet

Nutrition Grade A

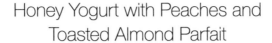

Honey Yogurt with Peaches and Toasted Almond Parfait

1 cup Fage Total Honey 2 percent Greek yogurt

⅓ cup toasted almonds

¾ cup sliced peaches (or cubed for small children)

In a large glass, layer half of the yogurt, half of the toasted almonds, and half of the fruit. Repeat the layers.

Serves 1

To toast almonds:

In a skillet, place nuts in an even layer and cook over medium heat, shaking often—don't overcrowd your nuts.

Keep stirring for about 5 minutes, or until nuts are fragrant and browned.

NUTRITION FACTS

Serving Size 128g	Amount Per Serving	
Calories 50	**Calories from Fat 3**	
		Daily Value*
Total Fat	0.3g	0%
Cholesterol	0mg	0%
Sodium	0mg	0%
Total Carbohydrates	12.2g	4%

Dietary Fiber	1.9g	8%
Sugars	10.7g	
Protein	1.2g	

Vitamin A 8% • Vitamin C 14% • Calcium 1% • Iron 2%

* Based on a 2000 calorie diet

Nutrition Grade A

Orange Almond Creamsicle

1½ cups orange juice

2 tbsp honey

1 cup low-fat vanilla frozen yogurt

½ cup almond milk

1 tsp vanilla extract

Combine the juice, honey, frozen yogurt, almond milk, and vanilla extract in a blender and blend until smooth. Pour into Popsicle molds and freeze until firm, about 10 hours.

To remove the pops from the molds, run under warm water to loosen.

NOTE: If you do not have Popsicle molds, try using Dixie cups and Popsicle sticks. Pour the mixture into Dixie cups, place in the freezer, and after four to six hours place Popsicle sticks into the center of each cup and continue to freeze for at least an additional six hours.

Yields 8–10 servings, depending on the size of your molds

NUTRITION FACTS

Serving Size 67g   Amount Per Serving

Calories 73   Calories from Fat 33

		Daily Value*
Total Fat	3.7g	6%
Saturated Fat	3.2g	16%
Cholesterol	0mg	0%
Sodium	3mg	0%
Total Carbohydrates	10.1g	3%
Sugars	8.8g	
Protein	0.7g	

Vitamin A 2% • Vitamin C 40% • Calcium 1% • Iron 2%

* Based on a 2000 calorie diet

Nutrition Grade C

Strawberry Clouds

Clouds

5 egg whites

1½ cups sweetener (Splenda)

1 tsp salt

½ tsp vanilla

Strawberry filling

1 pt strawberries, trimmed and sliced

2 tbsp sugar or sweetener

2 tsp vanilla

Preheat oven to 400°F.

Combine strawberries with sugar and vanilla; place in refrigerator and allow to marinate.

Beat egg whites until frothy. Add sweeter slowly and beat until stiff peaks form; adding salt and vanilla, continue to beat to maintain stiff peaks.

With a large spoon place 8 nest clouds on a cookie sheet that has been greased and lined with greased wax paper.

Bake until golden brown, remove from oven. Slice off toasted tops.

Spoon strawberries into meringue clouds and serve. These tasty desserts are fat free.

Serves 8

NUTRITION FACTS

Serving Size 106g   Amount Per Serving

Calories 220   **Calories from Fat 2**

		Daily Value*
Total Fat	0.2g	0%
Cholesterol	0mg	0%
Sodium	326mg	14%
Total Carbohydrates	42.9g	14%
Dietary Fiber	0.9g	4%
Sugars	41.6g	
Protein	2.5g	

Vitamin A 0% • Vitamin C 44% • Calcium 1% • Iron 1%

* Based on a 2000 calorie diet

Nutrition Grade D

Walnut Orange Shortbread

¼ cup walnuts

¾ cup all-purpose flour

½ cup whole-wheat flour

⅔ cup confectioners' sugar

½ tsp salt

½ cup (1 stick) unsalted butter, melted

¼ tsp vanilla

2 tbsp light olive or canola oil

2 tsp finely grated orange zest

1 tsp freshly squeezed orange juice

Preheat oven to 350°F.

Butter and flour two 8-inch round cake pans; set aside. In a food processor, combine nuts, flours, sugar, and salt; pulse until nuts are finely ground but not oily. Add the butter, vanilla, oil, orange zest, and orange juice; pulse until the mixture just comes together.

Divide the mixture between the two pans and press in until even. With a sharp knife, cut each round of dough into 8 wedges. Lightly prick the tops with the tines of a fork.

Bake until set and pale tan, about 22 minutes.

Transfer to a wire rack and cut through each wedge. Cool 10 minutes, then invert onto a plate and transfer to a wire rack to cool completely.

True You

Serves 16

NUTRITION FACTS

Serving Size 26g

Amount Per Serving

Calories 134

Calories from Fat 79

		Daily Value*
Total Fat	8.8g	13%
Saturated Fat	3.9g	19%
Trans Fat	0.0g	
Cholesterol	15mg	5%
Sodium	115mg	5%
Total Carbohydrates	12.7g	4%
Sugars	5.0g	
Protein	1.5g	

Vitamin A 4% • Vitamin C 1% • Calcium 0% • Iron 3%

* Based on a 2000 calorie diet

Nutrition Grade D
